SOUTH BEACH DIET FOR BEGINNERS

The Quickest, Safest, and Easiest Way to Lose Weight

(The Able Guide to Help Reverse Your Body Metabolism and Improve Your Health)

Cameron Brown

Published by Alex Howard

South Beach Diet for Beginners: The Quickest, Safest, and Easiest Way to Lose Weight (The Able Guide to Help Reverse Your Body Metabolism and Improve Your Health)

ISBN 978-1-77485-017-6

Legal & Disclaimer

The information contained in this book is not designed to replace or take the place of any form of medicine or professional medical advice. The information in this book has been provided for educational and entertainment purposes only.

Table of contents

Part 1 1

INTRODUCTION 2

Appetizers 55

Strawberry-Blueberry Crunch 55

Sweet Blueberry Fool 57

Crustless Mini Broccoli Quiche 59

Apple Cinnamon Granola cereal 61

Beach Shack Strawberry Shake 63

Salads 65

Broccoli-and-Cannellini Bean Salad 66

Red Bean Salad with Feta and Peppers 68

Kale Salad 70

Rainbow Raita 72

Black Bean and Corn Salad 74

Soups.. 76

Spicy Red Lentil Soup 76

Cauliflower Mushroom Chili....................... 79

Sweet Potato Black Bean Chili.................... 81

Broccoli and Cheese Soup 83

Cream of Broccoli Soup 85

Poultry and Meat 87

Jambalaya.. 87

Meat Loaf with Vegetables 89

Thai Grilled Beef with String Beef 91

Roasted Chicken Pomodoro 93

Broccoli and Cheese stuffed chicken breast...... 95

Spicy Buffalo and Asparagus with Miracle Noodles 97

Fish and Seafood 100

Cajun Shrimp with Steamed Cabbage 100

Grilled Shrimp and Raab............................. 103

Sweet Potato Tuna Patties 105

Foil Baked Fish... 107

Tender Juicy Lemon Baked Cod Recipe 109

DESSERTS 111

Chocolate Cake with Peanut Butter Frosting .. 111

Jeremy's Apple Puree 114

Jeremy's Cocoa Delight- Cocoa Crack............. 116

Chocolate Cream Cheese Cupcakes 118

Carrot-Pineapple Muffins............................. 120

CONCLUSION.. 122

Part 2 123

Introduction 124

Chapter 1: What is the South Beach Diet? 126

Chapter 2: The Truth About Carbs in the Body ... 135

Chapter 3: The 3 Phases in South Beach Diet and Foods Allowed in Each One 141

Chapter 4: Recipes During Phase 1 of the South Beach Diet 151

Vegetable Hash 151

Quiche Cups 152

Green Gazpacho 153

Tomato Soup 154

White Bean Soup 155

Labne Balls 156

Skillet Cod 157

Tomato and Spinach Salmon 158

Pecan Trout 159

Ginger Tenderloin 161

Shepherd's Pie 162

Veggie Chili 164

Potato Salad 165

Red Bean Mash 166

Baked Ricotta Custard 167

Chapter 5: Recipes for Phase 2 of the South Beach Diet 168

Egg Frijoles 168

Oat Muffins 170

Eggsadilla 172

Thai Shrimp Soup 173

Roasted Tomato Soup 174

Turkey Sausage Soup............................... 175

Florentine Soup 176

Stuffed Chicken Breast 177

Chicken and Soba Noodles 178

Herbed Turkey..................................... 180

Halibut and Vegetable Ragout 181

Shrimp and Scallop Bake 182

Stir-fry with Beef 184

Lamb Stew... 185

Barley Risotto 187

Sweet Potato Chips 188

Chapter 6: Recipes for Phase 3 of the South Beach Diet... 189

Classic Burger 189

Steak Wraps 190

Conclusion... 191

Part 1

INTRODUCTION

The South Beach Diet was originally a diet plan outlined in a book by Arthur Agatston, MD. The doctor developed the plan in the 1990s to help his patients lose weight. The South Beach Diet: The Delicious, Doctor-Designed, Foolproof Plan for Fast and Healthy Weight Loss flew off shelves in 2003 when it was first published.

Dr. Agatston noticed that patients on the Atkins diet were losing weight and abdominal fat. Being a cardiologist, he was concerned by the amount of saturated fat on Atkins, so he developed his own high-protein, low-carb diet that is lower in saturated fat.

Since that time, the book has gone through several variations and changes, but the core of the eating plan has stayed the same.

The South Beach Diet is a low-carb, high-protein and low-sugar program. The diet is based in part on the glycemic Index, which ranks foods according to glycemic load. As you learn how to do the South Beach Diet, you learn how to choose healthier, lower sugar foods to keep you full and satisfied so you eat less and slim down.

HOW IT WORKS

This diet focuses on a healthy balance between carbs, protein, and fat. More importantly, you are advised to consume high-quality carbohydrates, lean protein, and healthy fats. Foods with added sugars, like baked goods, sweets, and soft drinks are off limits. So if you are used to filling up on these foods, the diet may be hard to follow.

Prepackaged South Beach Diet foods, such as shakes, snack bars and prepared breakfast, lunch, and dinner meals are available for consumers who sign up for the paid program. Many of these foods are similar to foods that you may feel uncomfortable giving up. But you'll eat them in smaller quantities if you buy the South Beach versions and the foods are prepared with fewer calories.

The diet has three stages, known as phases, during which the proportion of carbohydrates is gradually increased, while the proportion of fats and protein are simultaneously decreased. The diet is comprised of a list of recommended foods such as lean meats, vegetables, and "good" (mostly monounsaturated) fats.

All three phases include specific allowable foods, meal plans, and recipes. Each phase also includes foods to avoid.

3

SOUTH BEACH DIET PHASE 1 (ALSO CALLED 7-DAY REBOOT)

For most people, the most difficult part of the program is Phase 1. In some versions of the plan, this phase lasted for two weeks. However, current versions of the use a 7-day "reboot" instead of a two-week phase.

This first part of the plan is the most stringent of the three phases. It is when you will limit the most carbs from your daily diet, including fruit, bread, rice, potatoes, pasta, sugar, alcohol, and baked goods.

The theory behind this phase is that there is a switch inside us that affects the way our bodies react to the food we eat and makes us gain weight. When the switch is on, we crave foods that actually cause us to store fat. However, by following the specified plan, you can correct the way your body reacts to food.

Many South Beach Diet fans swear that their cravings for sweets and other bad carbs virtually disappear during this reboot. For some, the first phase can be extended, but it is not meant to be a permanent way of eating.

SOUTH BEACH DIET PHASE 2

During this phase, you can start adding in more foods, such as additional sources of carbohydrates, like beans and legumes.

During Phase 2, the calorie range and the macronutrient breakdown are almost the same as in Phase 1 but the number of calories allowed from saturated fats decreases to less than 10 percent of total calories.

The exercise recommendation is to engage in at least 30 minutes of physical activity each day. Beginning in Phase 2 you can engage in more intense physical activity, if desired.

SOUTH BEACH DIET PHASE 3

Phase 3 is the final and least restrictive part of The South Beach Diet. Dr. Agatston says as long as you continue to follow some basic guidelines, the diet becomes your way of life and you'll continue to maintain your weight.

PROS AND CONS

Like any diet, the South Beach Diet has its own set of positives and negatives.

On the upside, the South Beach Diet is super simple and it encourages individual experimentation. When you sign up for the paid version of the program, you won't have to do any guesswork about portion sizes, and whether or not you pay for the program, the allowed and not allowed foods are clearly outlined.

On the other hand, the first portion of the South Beach Diet can seem extremely restrictive and potentially lead to disordered eating or yo-yo dieting down the road. Additionally, this diet promotes consumption of processed, packaged foods (the bars and shakes that come with the plan). The South Beach Diet may also not be structured enough in the later phases, which could result in weight regain for people who aren't sure how to control portion sizes after phases 1 and 2.

COMMON MYTHS AND QUESTIONS

Like many diets, several myths surround the South Beach Diet. Here are some common myths, and the truth that dispels them.

Myth: You can be successful on the South Beach Diet without exercise.

This is a loaded myth because it's true, but it isn't. Any diet regardless of types of food, timing and supplements can lead to weight loss as long as you're in a calorie deficit. That is, you eat fewer calories than you burn. However, when you rely on diet only for weight loss, your progress will be slow at best. Adding in a few minutes of exercise each day can expedite your weight loss goals regardless of what diet you're on.

Myth: You can lose weight just by implementing the bars and shakes from South Beach Diet.

Many people believe that just replacing foods with the South Beach Diet official snacks and shakes will result in weight loss. Unfortunately, successful weight loss isn't that easy: You must pay attention to your total caloric intake and make sure you're burning more calories than you eat. While replacing full meals with bars and shakes may result in weight loss, once regular eating is implemented weight regain is likely to occur.

Myth: You'll lose all the weight you need during Phase 1 of the South Beach Diet.

It's common to use short, extremely restrictive periods as a sort of "crash course" for weight loss. However, it's much more sustainable to lose weight slowly over time. Healthy, safe, and sustainable weight loss is generally 1-2 pounds per week. Extreme weight fluctuation is typically a result of water loss and sometimes muscle loss. Extreme weight fluctuations is typically a result of water loss and sometimes muscle.

Also, by severely restricting your food consumption for one week, you might set yourself up for a binge at the end of the week. If you don't continue to monitor your intake, you'll gain back all the weight you lost.

HOW IT COMPARES

The South Beach Diet has been compared to several diets, including other popular ones such as the Atkins Diet. The South Beach Diet differs from other low-carb diets in that it does not require dieters to cut out carbohydrates entirely or even measure their intake.6 Here's how it compares to some diets and the federal dietary guidelines.

Atkins vs. South Beach Diet

The Atkins diet is another low-carbohydrate plan. The Atkins Diet was also developed by a doctor and has gone through many variations through the years. The South Beach Diet has been called a less-strict version of Atkins. Both Atkins and South Beach require you to go through a strict introductory phase. But during the later phases of South Beach, you are able to eat more carbohydrates and enjoy treats on occasion. Both the Atkins and South Beach Diet include maintenance programs for long-term health and well-being.

There are slight differences between the South Beach and the Atkins diet in the type of protein allowed on each plan. On the Atkins diet, cured meats that are higher in sodium (such as ham) are allowed but not recommended. On South Beach, consumers are advised to skip these meats entirely. Pork bacon is allowed on Atkins, while only turkey bacon is allowed on South Beach. Keep in mind that processed meats have been associated with overweight, obesity, and increased risk of heart disease and cancer.

There are also slight differences in the types of dairy included on each plan. Atkins includes small portions of butter and heavy cream on their plan. While South Beach does not. Both diets recommend many full fat dairy products.

Keto vs. South Beach Diet

A keto diet is higher in fat and lower in protein than the South Beach diet. However, the introductory phase of the South Beach Diet is comparable in some ways to a ketogenic, or keto, diet. The difference is that the South Beach Diet becomes less strict as you work your way through the phases, allowing you to add in more carbohydrates. On a keto diet, however, the intention is to remain low-carb for the long haul.

Federal Recommendations vs South Beach Diet

The first two phases of the South Beach Diet don't match the federal dietary recommendations, which emphasize whole grains. However, the entire South Beach Diet emphasizes fiber-rich vegetables, fruits and lean protein, as well as minimal saturated fat and sugar. The South Beach Diet also outlines healthy exercise recommendations, which are close to the federal exercise recommendations for adults.

The first week of any new way of eating can be challenging. Know that there will be rough spots, especially as your body gets used to foods that weren't previously in your meal rotation as often, or cooked in that particular way, or ever. Give yourself compassion if you make inadvertent mistakes, and stay enthusiastic about your transformation. Remember that these nutritious foods are meant to improve your health and whittle your waistline. And If you have any pre-exisiting health conditions or are pregnant or nursing, this diet may not be right for you. Always consult with a healthcare provider before starting any diet plan.

WHAT TO EXPECT ON THE SOUTH BEACH DIET

The South Beach Diet touts many benefits, including substantial weight loss, stabilized blood sugar, reduced cravings, and increased energy. When following the South Beach Diet, you can expect a drastic change to your diet, at least in the first phase.

There are three phases of the South Beach Diet. Phase 1 is the most restrictive (no fruit, grains, starches, or alcohol) and lasts one to two weeks to help your body reboot and get used to burning fat instead of carbs for fuel. After that, you'll be able to slowly add foods with carbohydrates back into your diet.

WHAT TO EAT
Compliant Foods (Phase 1)

- Lean meats and poultry
- Eggs and egg whites
- Seafood
- Soy products
- Non-starchy vegetables
- Some beans
- Nuts
- Dairy
- Healthy fats

Non-Compliant Foods (Phase 1)

- Fatty cuts of meat
- Starchy vegetables
- Fruit
- Grains and starches
- Alcohol
- Sugar-sweetened beverages
- Desserts

It's important to note that the South Beach Diet includes three phases, and the foods you can and cannot eat differ as you move through the phases. Here's a rundown of what you can and can't eat during phases one, two and three.

13

PHASE 1

During Phase 1 of the South Beach Diet, you will be able to eat many of the foods you currently enjoy, including ground beef and a variety of vegetables. These foods are low on the glycemic index and are supposed to help you to eliminate cravings for starchy carbohydrates and sweets.

You'll cut carbohydrates during this phase, and that will help you to reduce excess water weight. You may see a five-pound change on the scale or even more in the span of a week.

Compliant Foods (Phase 1)

During Phase 1, these are the foods and ingredients you can incorporate into your diet:

- **Meats and poultry**

You can enjoy a range of protein sources on the South Beach Diet, as long as you focus on meats low in fat, especially saturated fats. Enjoy boiled ham, lean cuts of beef, such as flank steak or eye of round, skinless turkey and chicken breast, Canadian and turkey bacon, pork tenderloin, lower-fat and lower-sodium lunch meats including lean deli roast beef or smoked turkey.

- **Seafood**

You can eat all types of fish seafood on the South Beach Diet, but try to limit your intake of high-mercury fish and seafood.

- **Eggs**

The South Beach Diet permits whole eggs and egg whites, so you can still enjoy your morning omelet.

- **Soy products**

If you're vegetarian or vegan, you can opt for soy-based meat substitutes such as soy bacon or soy crumbles.

- **Beans**

Beans are a great source of fiber and plant-based protein, and you can eat many varieties on the South Beach Diet, including black-eyed peas, great northern beans, chickpeas, and pinto beans.

- **Nuts**

Snack on nuts such as almonds, cashews, and macadamia nuts, but you must limit your intake to one serving per day.

- **Non-starchy vegetables**

Any non-starchy vegetable is a go on the South Beach Diet. Incorporate a lot of leafy greens, sprouts, lettuce, okra, peppers, and cruciferous veggies like broccoli.

- **Dairy**

You're encouraged to enjoy full-fat dairy rather than low- or no-fat, because many manufacturers add sugar to make up for the lost flavor in low-fat options.

- **Healthy fats**

Each day, you can consume up to 2 tablespoons of healthy oils like olive oil; avocado (1/3 avocado equals one tablespoon of your healthy oil intake); and 2 tablespoons of salad dressing with less than 3 grams of sugar.

Non-compliant Foods (Phase 1)

Here's what you'll want to avoid:

- **Fatty cuts of meat**

You should avoid fatty meats like brisket and prime rib, dark meat from poultry, poultry with skin, duck meat, and chicken wings and legs. You should also avoid sugary meats such as honey-baked ham and beef jerky.

- **Starchy vegetables**

During Phase 1 of the South Beach Diet, you should avoid starchy vegetables such as potatoes and sweet potatoes, corn, beets, yams, turnips, and green peas.

- **Grains and starches**

You can't eat any carbohydrates from grain sources during Phase 1. This includes bread, crackers, chips, pretzels, oatmeal, cereal, pasta, granola, rice, bagels, buns, and other sources.

- **Alcohol**

Alcohol including beer, hard liquor, wine, and mixed drinks is off-limits during phase one.

- **Sugar-sweetened beverages**

Sports drinks, energy drinks, sodas, juices, and other beverages that contain sugar aren't allowed on the South Beach Diet. Ideally, you should also avoid artificially sweetened beverages as they can contribute to bloating and digestive discomfort.

- **Desserts**

Refrain from eating cookies, cakes, ice cream, candy, frozen yogurt, and other sugary desserts during Phase 1 of the South Beach Diet.

PHASE 2

Compliant Foods (Phase 2)

- Everything in Phase 1, plus:
- Starchy vegetables
- Whole grains
- Fruit

Non-Compliant Foods (Phase 2)

- Fatty cuts of meat
- Sugar-sweetened beverages
- Alcohol
- Desserts

In the first two weeks on South Beach, you eat from a list of foods, and that's it. After the first phase, it's time to start individualizing the diet for your own body and tastes.

The goal of Phase 2 of the South Beach Diet is to find the right carb level for you. This is done by gradually reintroducing some high nutrient, high fiber, low glycemic carbohydrates into your diet. How much and what types will vary between individuals. During this phase, weight loss will likely slow to one to two pounds per week, so keep this in mind as well.

Phase 2 of the South Beach Diet lasts until you reach your goal weight.

Week One

The plan of the first week of Phase 2 is to add one serving of a carbohydrate food to each day, experimenting to see how you feel. Chances are this first food will not be problematic.

What should the food be? Generally, it is a serving from the approved fruit list or a serving of a low-glycemic starch. Dr. Arthur Agatson, the creator of the South Beach Diet, recommends that if you choose fruit to have it at lunch or dinner. He thinks that fruit at breakfast is more likely to induce cravings.

If you choose an approved whole grain, he recommends a high fiber, low-carb cereal such as Fiber One, All Bran with extra fiber, or slow-cooked oatmeal (not instant). If you are having cereal for breakfast, be sure to include some protein as well.

Week Two

In the second week, you will add a second daily serving of carbohydrate food, as above. That means you will be eating one serving of fruit and one serving of a high-fiber starchy food each day this week, in addition to all the other foods.

Week Three

During the third week, you will again add a serving of carbohydrate food daily if you can tolerate it without weight gain or cravings. It's also probably a good idea to talk a bit about bread at this point. Look for bread with at least 3 grams of fiber per serving—bread made specifically to be low-carb usually has more fiber and less starch. If bread is a problem for you, at this point or later, choose a grain that is not ground into flour, such as brown rice, and see if you tolerate it better.

Week Four

Add another serving of carbohydrates. At this point, you may be getting near the limit of carbohydrates you can eat and continue to lose weight and some people will have passed that limit. Watch carefully for the signs of carb cravings.

Week Five

If you can handle it, add another serving of carbohydrates. At this point, your menus should look like Phase 1 meals but with the addition of two or three servings each of fruit, starches or grains, and dairy. Lunch and dinner should each have at least 2 cups of vegetables along with a serving of protein.

Week Six

If you are still able to add carbohydrates, you will be eating three servings of fruit and three servings of grains or starches. If this is too much carbohydrate, try substituting more non-starchy vegetables. At this point, you have transitioned completely into Phase 2 of the South Beach Diet. This is the way you should eat until you reach your goal weight and are ready for Phase 3.

PHASE 3

Compliant Foods (Phase 3)

- Everything in Phase 2, plus:
- More grains
- More variety from all food groups

Non-Compliant Foods (Phase 3)

- Nothing is technically off-limits

You made your goal weight! Now what?

This is the lifelong endpoint of the South Beach Diet. You have now attained your goal weight. But even more important for long-term success, you have learned to eat and enjoy healthier food. You can celebrate your success but you need to make the most of what you learned along the way.

What Can You Eat in Phase 3?

The short answer is that you can eat anything you want. But that depends on what you want to eat, and how much. You can't forget the lessons you learned in Phase 1 and 2, making better choices to enjoy lean protein, vegetables, healthy oils, and appropriate portions. Desserts, alcohol, sugary drinks, and fatty meats should remain off-limits for the best results.

You will be able to determine the number of carbs you can add back into your diet without gaining weight. If you see your weight increase, cut back on carbs. If you need to lose weight, you can start the Phases over again.

How Long to Follow Phase 3

By the time you reach Phase 3, you will have learned all the skills you need to maintain your goal weight, and you can maintain Phase 3 for good if you wish.

RECOMMENDED TIMING

The South Beach Diet doesn't enforce any specific timing for your meals or snacks. Rather, people on the diet are simply encouraged to eat up to six times per day: three meals, and three snacks, a pretty typical recommendation.

It's a good idea to space your meals and snacks out by two to four hours going too long without food can lead to hunger pangs, which can lead to overeating. Don't forget to drink plenty of water before, during, and after your meals. Staying hydrated will help you feel fuller for longer.

RESOURCES AND TIPS

If you're serious about losing weight and keeping it off on The South Beach Diet, you should download and print the South Beach Diet Handbook. This handbook includes a list of approved foods for every stage of the weight loss program, including weight maintenance.

Set Yourself Up for Success

If you're concerned that you won't be able to survive the first stage of the South Beach Diet, you're not alone. Many people find the list of Phase 1 foods to be too restrictive. But if you want to make the diet work, there are a few ways to set yourself up for success:

• **Fill your pantry with your favorite Phase 1 diet foods**

Get the complete list, find the foods that make you most happy, and fill your kitchen with those items. Schedule an hour (at least) to visit the grocery store and check out areas of the market that you generally skip. You might find new foods and flavors to explore.

• **Clean out your kitchen**

Make sure all foods that are not allowed are thrown away. That means that you clean out your refrigerator and pantry and set up your kitchen for weight loss success. Having the wrong foods in your kitchen will only make the first phase more difficult.

- **Start the South Beach Diet exercise plan**

You'll be less likely to crave the Phase 1 diet foods you can't eat if you fill your day with healthy activity that gets you away from the kitchen. The South Beach exercise program is specifically designed for beginners who want to burn calories and stay active. And if you follow the plan precisely, you won't do too much too soon and get hungry or tired as a result.

Phase 1 Tips

Once you know which foods to eat and which foods to avoid during Phase 1 of the South Beach Diet, use these helpful tips to eat better and lose weight.

- **Don't rely on "healthy" foods**

Just because a food is healthy, doesn't mean that it is good for your diet during Phase 1. In fact, many healthy foods are not allowed during Phase 1 of the South Beach Diet. Fruit is a good example. Whole fruit contains fiber and other healthy vitamins and minerals. But because fruit contains a lot of sugar (fructose) it is not allowed during Phase 1. Homemade baked goods are another food to ditch during Phase 1. Stick to the food list to make meal and snack choices—even when the menu options sound healthy.

- **Stick to unprocessed foods**

The tricky thing about Phase 1 is that you have to avoid certain foods like sugar but also any product that contains that food as an ingredient. If you eat heavily processed packaged foods, you'll have to scour the ingredients list of every product you buy to uncover hidden ingredients. It's easier and healthier to eat whole foods in their natural state.

- **Measure portion sizes**

Portion size matters on every diet. It is especially important during Phase 1 of The South Beach diet if you want to lose a lot of weight. Many items on the Phase 1 food list have suggested serving sizes. Nuts, for example, are limited to one serving per day and each variety of nut has a different serving size. Only 2 cups of dairy products are allowed each day and sweet treats are limited to 75–100 calories per day.

Get creative in the kitchen. You'll be able to eat more food and you'll be less hungry if you cook your own healthy South Beach Diet foods. There are plenty of recipes online and in the book. Try new recipes and experiment with new flavors. It will help you to keep your mind off of the foods that are not allowed during Phase 1.

- **Plan meals and snacks in advance**

It's going to be natural to want to fall back into your old eating habits during Phase 1 of the South Beach Diet. In social situations and during stressful moments you're going to be tempted to reach for the foods that used to bring you comfort. So how do you combat those cravings? Be prepared. Plan your meals and snacks in advance so that you always have Phase 1 foods on hand.

Phase 2 Tips

You may want to keep a food journal during Phase 2 to set yourself up for success in Phase 3, when you no longer rely solely on food lists. You'll have much more control over what you eat, when, and how often.

If you learn as much as possible during Phase 2 about the foods that make you feel good, the foods that trigger cravings, and the foods you're tempted to overeat, you'll be more likely to continue your healthy South Beach Diet eating habits in a way that is satisfying and sustainable for long-term health.

Phase 3 Tips

You first will have gone through the restrictive food list in Phase 1, which cuts out most of the carbohydrates from your diet. This is a week-long phase to get you out of cravings for high-sugar foods. For many people, that is the bulk of their diet before they start the South Beach Diet, so it can be quite a hurdle to overcome.

But in the two weeks on Phase 1, you also learn to eat (and hopefully enjoy) healthier options. This re-education of your palate and change to your plate will be something you carry into Phase 2 and 3. lean protein, high-fiber vegetables, low-fat dairy products. Here you also learned to use unsaturated fats, nuts, seeds, and avocados.

You probably also re-educated yourself as to what a healthy food portion was, so you will know to look at a plate whether it contains more food than you should eat in one meal.

MODIFICATIONS

It is very important to pay attention to your own body's reactions to adding the carbs. If a food sets up cravings or weight gain, back off and try something less glycemic. If you feel fuzzy-headed or lower in energy, ditto.

As always, be attentive to your allergies and sensitivities. The South Beach Diet includes a relatively wide range of foods, especially after the first phase, so you should be able to swap foods as needed.

If cost is a factor for you, don't buy into the paid program. You can save money by buying your groceries and prepping food yourself. On the other hand, if convenience is a bigger factor for you than finances, the paid program with pre-portioned and delivered food may be a good option for you.

You shouldn't attempt Phase 1 if you have a history of disordered eating. Severe food restriction can lead to food fear and labeling of foods as "good" or "bad."

PROS AND CONS OF THE SOUTH BEACH DIET

The South Beach Diet is a popular diet that takes you through phases. During Phase 1, you'll cut out virtually all carbohydrates to get rid of bloat and "reboot" your body; during Phase 2, you'll slowly start adding carbohydrates back into your body; and by Phase 3, you're expected to have met your goal weight and learned new healthy eating habits.

The South Beach Diet claims to make you feel less hungry and contribute to a number of good health outcomes, including lower triglycerides and blood glucose; lower blood pressure, higher HDL, among others.

But like all diets, not everyone takes well to the South Beach Diet. Here we explain the positives and negatives of the diet and what sets it apart from other low-carb diets.

Pros

- Very simple
- Low in saturated fats
- Emphasizes healthy eating patterns
- Encourages individual experimentation
- Gives your body a chance to reset

Cons

- Very restrictive first phase
- Some inconsistencies
- No evidence for weight loss
- Possibly not enough structure
- May contribute to disordered eating

PROS OF THE SOUTH BEACH DIET

Overall, the South Beach Diet can be healthy and well-rounded, with the exception of the first phase, which restricts carbohydrate intake.

Simplicity

There's no counting and not much measuring on the South Beach Diet. For the most part, you just choose foods from certain lists and eat within that, so you won't have to deal with any guesswork or counting calories of each food.

Low in Saturated Fats

Low-carb diet authors have different opinions on whether it's important to limit saturated fats on reduced carb diets; however, no author recommends relying on them.

Encourages Individual Experimentation

One of the strongest aspects of the diet is the focus on each person being aware of the effects of foods on their bodies, particularly as they add carbohydrates. Using the marker of carb cravings can be a useful one, as it's vital for people who are sensitive to carbohydrates to be aware of what foods and what quantities trigger these cravings.

Gives Your Body a Chance to Reset

While we don't think fasting or restricting food groups is the best way to start any healthy eating program, a one-week reset does work well for many people. For example, you may have some food sensitivities you didn't know about, and Phase 1 of the South Beach Diet could help you uncover those.

Emphasizes Healthy Eating Patterns

After Phase 1 ends, the South Beach Diet is really all about creating sustainable and well-rounded eating patterns. The end goal does involve weight loss for most people, but South Beach emphasizes long-term healthy habits, and that's a goal we can get behind.

A successful version of the South Beach Diet involves powering through the first phase and then slowly discovering how many carbohydrates (and what kinds) your body can handle. The South Beach Diet offers some positives that make it a great diet for some (e.g., those who value simplicity) but may not be the best choice for everyone.

CONS OF THE SOUTH BEACH DIET

Like most diets, the South Beach Diet presents some drawbacks, most of which revolve around its restrictive and difficult Phase 1.

Very Restrictive First Phase

The limitations of the first phase may be a real turn off for some people. On the other hand, it's short-term, and the author doesn't recommend anyone staying with it longer than 3 or 4 weeks at most (for people who have quite a bit of weight to lose). Since there are no guidelines as to how much carbohydrate to eat, "carb crash" could also occur, depending upon the individual dieter's food selections.

Some Inconsistencies

Quite a few aspects of the diet don't really fit together well. For example, more saturated fat is allowed in Phase 3, when a primary aspect in Phases 1 and 2 was to limit saturated fat. Additionally, the creator, Dr. Aruthur Agatston recommends some highly processed carbs, such as couscous, and has many recipes which include it. Other high-glycemic foods are in his menus and recipes, which may send, at the least, a mixed message.

No Evidence for Weight Loss

The South Beach Diet markets itself as a weight-loss solution, but there's no solid evidence to uphold that claim. According to a study published in 2016, there is evidence that low-carb diets support weight loss, but South Beach doesn't stay low-carb for long, so that relationship doesn't pan out, either. There is little research on the South Beach diet, however a study published in 2014 suggested that it isn't any more effective than other commercial diets, and is especially ineffective at promoting long-term weight loss.

Possibly Not Enough Structure

For some people, there may not be enough structure when it comes to adding carbs back in. This diet leaves a lot up to the individual, which is good in the long run but is probably harder in the short run. Also, some people just aren't all that tuned into their bodies' signals and might not be motivated to become so.

Can Be Expensive

You can follow the South Beach principles on your own, but if you opt to participate in the paid program and get meals delivered to your door, expect to pay a few hundred dollars per month for the convenience.

May Contribute to Disordered Eating

Any diet that labels foods as "good" and "bad" hold the potential to result in disordered eating and an unhealthy relationship with food. Because the South Beach Diet places such an emphasis on "good" and "bad" carbohydrate sources and fats, it may lead to food fear.

In the end, whether or not you should try the South Beach Diet comes down to personal preference and your goals. You should start a diet for the right reasons, and South Beach might be right for you if:

•   You want to uncover food sensitivities to carbohydrate sources
•   You want a one-week "reboot" that may help you feel better without too severely restricting calorie intake
•   You want to learn more about your body and what a healthy eating pattern looks like for you

The South Beach Diet may not be for you if:

•   You're solely in it for weight loss (there's no solid evidence to support this)
•   You have a history of disordered eating or an unhealthy relationship with food or your body

- You're very active: lack of carbohydrates may affect your athletic performance or lead to hypoglycemia

SOUTH BEACH DIET VS. OTHER DIETS

The South Beach Diet is an interesting eating plan because it emphasizes both foods that we know to be healthy, such as leafy greens, as well as foods we know to be harmful, such as certain vegetable oils.

It's advertised as a low-carb diet, but it doesn't cut out all carbohydrates and it's much lower in fat than most low-carb diets such as the keto diet. Instead, the focus is on eating low-glycemic carbohydrates and lots of lean protein, which is thought to stabilize blood sugar, reduce cravings and promote weight loss.

The 2019 U.S. News and World Report Best Diets ranks the South Beach Diet number 20 in Best Diets Overall and gives it an overall score of 3.1/5.

USDA GUIDELINES

Compared to the USDA Dietary Guidelines for Americans, the South Beach Diet lacks in some ways but it doesn't stray too far from the federal suggestions. The USDA Dietary Guidelines Key Recommendations include:

- A variety of vegetables from all of the subgroups—dark green, red and orange, legumes (beans and peas), starchy vegetables
- Fruits, especially whole fruits
- Grains, at least half of which are whole grains
- Fat-free or low-fat dairy, including milk, yogurt, cheese, and/or fortified soy beverages
- A variety of protein foods, including seafood, lean meats and poultry, eggs, legumes (beans and peas), and nuts, seeds, and soy products
- Oils
- Limited saturated fats, trans fats, added sugars and sodium

Food Groups

In Phase 1, the South Beach Diet restricts virtually all carbohydrates, including fruits and whole grains, but Phase 1 only lasts for 14 days. Phase 2 begins on the 15th day, at which point, you can start incorporating small portions of fruit and "good carbs" back into your diet. From there, the South Beach Diet is mostly congruent with the USDA Guidelines, emphasizing whole grains, vegetables, fruits, lean protein, and healthy fats.

Overall, the South Beach Diet encourages a higher fat intake and a lower carbohydrate intake than the federal recommendations. Your protein consumption on South Beach would be cohesive with the USDA Dietary Guidelines.

Calories

Hunger shouldn't be an issue on the South Beach Diet. While the diet doesn't specify a calorie count that will depend on your current body weight, goal weight, and when you want to reach your goal weight it does encourage strategic snacking to dampen hunger before it strikes.

In fact, the South Beach Diet encourages you not to count calories, and instead focus on the types of food you eat. That said, you still need to pay attention to your caloric intake if your ultimate goal is weight loss. To lose weight, you must burn more calories than you eat.

Here's a helpful calorie calculator to help you find out how many calories you need each day to reach your goal.

Variety

The South Beach Diet actually does a great job of incorporating variety, especially in the later phases. You'll still be able to eat a range of satiating foods on the South Beach Diet that should satisfy both your physiological hunger cues and social or emotional cues, i.e., cravings.

The South Beach Diet encourages you to eat plenty of vegetables and get your protein from different sources, so you may actually end up eating more variety than you ever did before.

SIMILAR DIETS

The South Beach Diet is primarily a low-carb diet, so you can liken it to a few other popular low-carb diets.

ATKINS DIET

Like the South Beach Diet, the Atkins Diet was developed by a physician (Dr. Robert Atkins) who wanted to help his patients lose weight. Atkins also has phases like the South Beach Diet.

General Nutrition

Atkins advises eating a variety of fats, including saturated, polyunsaturated, and monounsaturated fat, whereas South Beach emphasizes the minimal intake of saturated fats from sources such as butter. Your food choices are more limited on the Atkins Diet than on the South Beach Diet, so you may be able to reach the USDA Dietary Guidelines recommendations more easily on South Beach.

Cost/Accessibility

Atkins and South Beach both provide a wealth of resources for people who follow their diets. Both websites detail a great deal of information, and you can find books on both diets. As far as cost goes, both meal plans can be pretty pricey. You can expect to pay a few hundred dollars per month to follow the plans to a T. However, you don't need to purchase the paid program for either diet in order to follow the guidelines.

Weight Loss

There's more research on the Atkins Diet than there is on The South Beach Diet, but both have been found to contribute to moderate weight loss.

Sustainability

Both diets require you to give up many foods that you may be used to eating, particularly the South Beach Diet in the beginning. Overall, though, the South Beach Diet is more flexible and doesn't require as much tracking as Atkins does.

NUTRISYSTEM

General Nutrition

Nutrisystem actually owns South Beach, so it makes sense that their approaches are similar. Like South Beach, Nutrisystem revolves around the glycemic index, but this program doesn't cut out carbs. Instead, Nutrisystem focuses on a high-protein diet with "good" carbs, such as vegetables and whole grains that fill you up with fiber.

Cost/Accessibility

On the Nutrisystem program, you'll eat the company's pre-packaged, delivered meals and snacks, plus some products you buy on your own. But the convenience and ease of the program comes at a price: A four-week plan starts at $10.54 each day, plus more if you want greater variety and extra shakes. On top of that, you'll still have to buy your own kitchen essentials, such as milk, fruit, and other items.

Weight Loss

Nutrisystem's core claim is that you can lose up to 13 pounds and 7 inches in your first month. There's some research that suggests you'll lose weight with Nutrisystem, but the majority of said research is company-funded, so there's a conflict of interest.

Sustainability

Because you'll be outsourcing a lot of your shopping, meal preparation, and cooking, you'll find that following Nutrisystem is easy. In that sense, the program is sustainable, and even more so because it's not necessarily restrictive.

WEIGHT WATCHERS DIET

General Nutrition

Weight Watchers takes a different approach than most diets: On Weight Watchers, no foods are off-limits. Because of this, Weight Watchers can be much more well-rounded than other diets, as it allows you to include foods from all of the food groups. Also, the focus is on a healthy lifestyle rather than just weight loss.

Cost/Accessibility

Weight Watchers can be pricey to participate in because it uses a membership model that includes access to weight loss and lifestyle coaches. To join, you pay an initial fee and then a monthly fee that differs based on the type of membership you chose.

Weight Loss

Most studies on Weight Watchers confirm that it's a good way to lose weight, especially in the short-term.

One study suggests that Weight Watchers is more effective at promoting sustained weight loss than other diets.

Sustainability

Due to its "points" approach, Weight Watchers can be very sustainable. You can eat whatever you want, as long as you stick to your daily SmartPoints target, a number calculated using your gender, weight, height, and age.

KETO DIET

General Nutrition

On a traditional ketogenic diet, you'll consume less than five percent of your total calories from carbohydrate for the long haul. The South Beach Diet, on the other hand, only restricts carbohydrates for a short period of time and then allows you to slowly reintroduce them. So in the long run, South Beach is more well-rounded.

Cost/Accessibility

A keto diet isn't a commercial diet; rather, it's just an overarching way of eating, so you won't have to purchase any special plan to eat a keto diet. That said, you don't need to buy the South Beach Diet program to be successful there, either. Many foods on both diets can get pricey, for example, avocados and olive oil.

Weight Loss

Some research has shown that keto promotes weight loss,7 but other research has shown that a keto diet is no more effective than a low-fat diet or other low-carb programs.7 When it comes to weight loss, the best diet is the one you can stick to.

Sustainability

Many people have trouble sticking to keto because it's very restrictive and not like the typical American diet. The South Beach Diet may be easier to stick to because the restrictive phase is short.

PALEO DIET

General Nutrition

The paleo diet is similar to the South Beach Diet because both encourage you to eat meat (preferably grass-fed), seafood, vegetables, eggs, nuts/seeds, and healthy oils. You'll keep your carb intake low on the paleo diet and refrain from eating bread, pasta, cereal or other grain-based foods, similar to Phase 1 of South Beach. However, one important thing to note about the paleo diet is that no processed foods are allowed, and on South Beach, you're encouraged to eat prepackaged foods, such as shakes, that the company provides.

Cost/Accessibility

Unlike the South Beach Diet, the paleo diet isn't a commercial diet and you don't need to purchase a program. However, the foods encouraged by the paleo community can be expensive: Die-hard paleo advocates eat grass-fed beef, cage-free eggs, and organic produce.

Weight Loss

Some studies have shown the Paleo diet to aid in weight loss, but results have been inconsistent, as they have been with other diets.

Sustainability

The simple truth is that cutting carbs is hard. Not many people can stick to a carb-restrictive diet for the long haul, which means paleo might not be the right choice for some people.

Appetizers

Strawberry-Blueberry Crunch

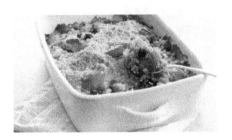

Preparation Time: 35 mins
Servings: 3
Ingredients:

- Whole almonds (1/4 cup)
- Sliced almonds(2 tbs)
- Freshly ground nutmeg (1/4 tsp)
- Ground cinnamon (1/4 tsp)
- Trans-fat-free margarine (1 tbs)
- Sliced strawberries (2 cups)
- Blueberries (1 cup)
- Granular sugar substitute (1 tbs)
- Part-skim ricotta cheese (6 tbs)

Directions:

1. Grind the whole almonds using a spice grinder until finely ground.
2. Combine the nutmeg, ground almonds, and cinnamon.
3. Add the margarine and stir to combine.
4. Coat the baking dish with cooking spray.
5. Place the sugar substitute and strawberries in the dish.
6. Dot using the ground nut mixture, then sprinkle using sliced almonds.
7. Bake for 35 minutes, until the fruit is hot or topping is golden.
8. Divide the fruit, and serve each bowl with a tablespoon of ricotta as topping.

Nutritional Facts
Per Serving:

Calories	100kCal
Fat	6g
Carbs	10g
Protein	4g
Fiber	3g
Sodium	35mg

Sweet Blueberry Fool

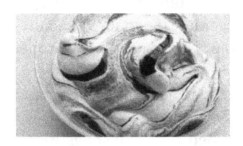

Preparation Time: 40 mins
Servings: 4
Ingredients:

- Fresh blueberries (1 pint) or frozen blueberries, not thawed (One 12-ounce bag)
- Granular sugar substitute (3 tbs)
- Fresh lime juice (2 tbs)
- Nonfat Greek-style yogurt
- Light or Fat-free whipped topping (1/2 cup)
- Four mint sprigs, for garnish

Directions:

1. Combine the lime juice, blueberries, 2 tablespoon of water, and sugar substitute in a saucepan.
2. Place the pan over medium heat and cook for 10 minutes, stirring continuously until the blueberries are soft.

3. Press the mixture through a fine strainer to remove the skin.

4. Transfer the contents to a container, cover and let it cool in a refrigerator for about 20 minutes.

5. Combine the yogurt and whipped topping in a medium bowl.

6. Fold in the blueberry puree gently, leaving a swirly pattern of the puree in the cream.

7. Serve garnished with mint sprigs.

Nutritional Facts

Per Serving:

Calories	104kCal
Fat	2g
Carbs	17g
Protein	5g
Fiber	2g
Sodium	22mg

Crustless Mini Broccoli Quiche

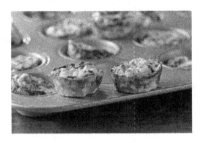

Preparation Time: 30 mins
Servings: 8
Ingredients:

- Broccoli florets (1/2 pound)
- Four eggs
- Milk (1 cup)
- Chopped Onion (1/2 cup)
- Grated cheese (1/2 cup)
- Salt (1 tsp)
- Pepper (1 tsp)

Directions:

1. On each muffin fold, place 1-2 florets, depending on the sides, and set aside.
2. Beat the milk and eggs until almost frothy, then add pepper and salt and mix well.

3. Pour this mixture into the muffin molds, just enough to cover the florets, then top each mold with grated cheese. Ensure that you leave enough space because the quiche may rise during baking.

4. Bake at 375 F for approximately 20 minutes, until top is browned.

5. Serve and enjoy!

Nutritional Facts
Per Serving:

Calories	120kCal
Fat	7g
Cholesterol	99mg
Sodium	432mg
Carbs	4g
Protein	8g

Apple Cinnamon Granola cereal

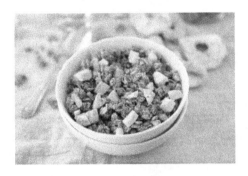

Preparation Time: 5 mins
Serving: 1
Ingredients:

- Whole grain rolled oats
- Soy Protein crisp
- Chicory root fiber
- Dried apples
- Salt
- Cane sugar
- Cinnamon
- Monk fruit juice concentrate
- Whey protein isolate
- Soy protein crisp
- Natural flavors
- Citric acid
- Milk (1/2 cup)

Directions:

1. Combine all the ingredients into a bowl, then add the milk.

2. Serve and enjoy.

Nutritional Facts

Per serving:

Calories	125kCal
Fat	1g
Sodium	125mg
Sugars	4g
Protein	10g
Calcium	64mg
Iron	2mg
Potassium	90mg

-

Beach Shack Strawberry Shake

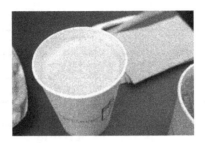

Preparation Time: 10 mins
Servings: 2
Ingredients:

- Sunflower oil
- Natural flavor
- Agave powder
- Salt
- Guar gum
- Calcium Caseinate from Milk
- Monk fruit extract
- Beet and sweet potato powder
- Water

Directions:
1. Add a cup of water, and a 1/2 cup of ice to a shaker bottle.
2. Toss in the contents of the powder packs, then screw the lid and shake vigorously to dissolve the powders.

3. Serve and enjoy!

Nutritional Facts
Per serving:

Calories	190kCal
Fat	10g
Cholesterol	5mg
Carbs	16g
Sodium	410mg
Fiber	2g
Protein	10g

Salads

Broccoli-and-Cannellini Bean Salad

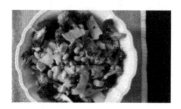

Preparation Time: 10 mins
Servings: 3

Ingredients:

- Coarsely chopped broccoli florets (1 1/2 cups)
- Red wine vinegar (2 tbs)
- Extra-virgin olive oil (2 tsp)
- Pepper (1/4 tsp)
- Salt (1/8 tsp)
- One Minced garlic cloves
- Finely chopped, bottled and roasted red bell pepper or chopped pimento (1/4 cup)
- Finely chopped red onion (1/4 cup)
- Cannellini beans (One 15-ounce can). or white bens rinsed and drained
- Lettuce leaves

Directions:
1. Steam the broccoli and cover the pot for 3 minutes, until the broccoli is crisp-tender, then set it aside.
2. Mix the oil, garlic, salt, and vinegar in a medium bowl as you toss the ingredients gently.
3. Serve on lettuce and enjoy!

Nutritional Facts

Per Serving:

Calories	129kCal
Fat	3.6g
Protein	6.2g
Carbs	18.1g
Fiber	1.8g
Iron	2.1mg
Sodium	266mg
Calcium	48mg

Red Bean Salad with Feta and Peppers

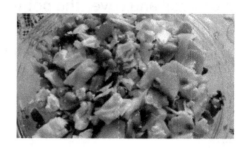

Preparation Time: 20 mins
Servings: 3
Ingredients:

- Kidney beans (One 15-ounce can)
- 1 chopped red bell pepper
- Chopped cabbage (2 cups)
- 2 green onions
- Crumbled feta cheese (1 cup)
- Fresh, chopped parsley (1/3 cup)
- 1 minced garlic cloves
- Lemon juice (2 tbs)
- Olive oil (1 tbs)

Directions:
1. Combine the beans, cabbage, red pepper, feta, garlic, parsley, onions, olive oil, and lemon juice, then cover and refrigerate for up to 3 days.

Nutritional Facts

Per Serving:

Calories	245kCal
Fat	12g
Carbs	23.8g
Protein	12.2g
Cholesterol	33mg
Sodium	658mg

Kale Salad

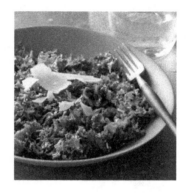

Preparation Time: 20 mins
Servings: 4-6
Ingredients:

- Extra-virgin olive oil (6 tbs)
- Red wine vinegar (2 tbs)
- 1 kale bunch, washed with stems removed
- 1 diced red cabbage head
- 1 bell pepper, diced into small chunks
- 1 chopped cilantro bunch
- 1 finely diced red onion

Directions:

1. Mix vinegar and oil together.
2. Toss the salad with dressing and let it chill in the refrigerator for 1 hour or so. This will allow the flavors to blend.

Nutritional Facts

Per Serving:

Calories	219kCal
Fat	21g
Carbs	9g
Protein	2g
Sodium	12mg
Fiber	2g

Rainbow Raita

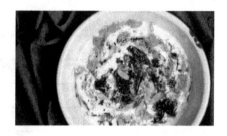

Preparation Time: 10 mins
Servings: 2
Ingredients:

- 1/2 cucumber, peeled and grated (1 cup)
- Low-fat plain yogurt (1 cup)
- Two grated, medium carrots (3/4 cup)
- 1/2 finely diced, red onions (1/2 cup)
- Chopped fresh mint (1/4 cup)

Directions:
Combine all ingredients in small bowl. Season to taste with salt and pepper, if desired.

Nutritional Facts
Per Serving:

Calories	31kCal
Protein	2g
Fat	1g
Carbs	5g
Cholesterol	2mg

Sodium	176mg
Fiber	1g
Sugars	3g

Black Bean and Corn Salad

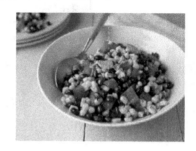

Preparation Time: 25 mins
Servings: 2
Ingredients:

- Fresh Lime juice (1/3 cup)
- Olive oil (1/2 cup)
- One minced garlic clove
- Salt (1 tsp)
- Ground cayenne pepper (1/8 tsp)
- Black beans, rinsed and drained (2 15-ounce can)
- Frozen corn kernels (1 1/2 cups)
- 1 peeled, pitted and diced avocado
- 1 chopped red bell pepper
- 2 chopped tomatoes
- 6 thinly sliced green onions
- Fresh, chopped cilantro (1/2 cup)

Directions:

1. Place the olive oil, lime juice, salt, garlic, and cayenne pepper in a small jar.
2. Cover the lid of the jar, and shake the jar until the ingredients are properly mixed.
3. Combine the corn, beans, bell pepper, avocado, green onions, tomatoes, and cilantro in a salad bowl.
4. Shake the lime dressing and pour it over the salad, and stir the salad to coat beans and vegetables with dressing.
5. Serve and enjoy!

Nutritional Facts

Per Serving:

Calories	391kCal
Fat	24.5g
Carbs	35.1g
Protein	10.5g
Sodium	830mg

Soups

Spicy Red Lentil Soup

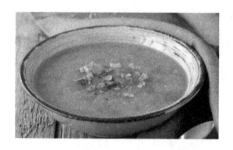

Preparation Time: 1 hr
Servings: 7
Ingredients:

- Water (4 cups)
- Goya Red lentils (1 cup)
- Margarine (2 tbs)
- 1/4-inch diced, peeled onions (1/2 cup)
- 1/2 Diced bell pepper
- 1/4-inch diced, trimmed celery (1/4 cup)
- Chopped garlic (2 tbs)
- Vegetable stock (2 cups)
- One medium tomato, cored and diced (approx. 1 cup)
- Hot sauce (1 tbs)
- Turmeric (1/8 tsp)
- Cumin (1/8 tsp)

- Cayenne pepper (1/8 tsp)
- Wegmans Sea Salt (1 tsp)
- Black pepper (1/2 tsp)
- Chili powder (1/8 tsp)

Directions:

1. Bring the lentils and water (2 cup) to boil on high heat then turn off the heat.
2. Remove half of the lentils and liquid, then place it in a blender/food processor and blend for about 1 min.
3. Melt the margarine in the stockpot on medium low heat, add the onions, and continue to cook as you stir for 2 more minutes, until they become soft. Ensure that they don't turn brown though.
4. Add the pepper, celery and garlic, and then continue to cook for 5 more minutes until soft. Add the tomato and let it cook for 5 minutes.
5. Add the rest of the remaining water, the stock, turmeric, Tabasco, pepper, and chili powder then bring the food to simmer.
6. Add the reserved whole and pureed lentil together with the liquid. Let it cook for 15 more minutes, until the lentils are tender.
7. Season with salt.

Nutritional Facts
Per Serving:

Calories	140kCal

Carbs	22g
Fiber	5g
Protein	7g
Fat	4g
Sat Fat	3g
Cholesterol	10mg
Sodium	410mg

Cauliflower Mushroom Chili

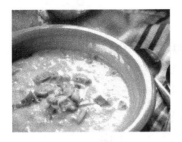

Preparation Time: 30 mins
Servings: 2
Ingredients:

- One diced sweet onion
- Three minced garlic cloves
- Fire roasted diced tomatoes (1 15-oz can)
- Apple cider vinegar (1 tbs)
- Chili powder (2 tbs)
- Ground cumin (1 tsp)
- dried oregano (1 tsp)
- Steak sauce (1 tbs)
- Yellow mustard (2 tsp)
- Curry powder (1/2 tsp)
- 1 head cauliflower, chopped bite size

Directions:

1. Pulse the mushrooms in a food processor until crumbled.
2. In a large pot, pour in the broth, mushrooms, garlic, and onions, and cook over high heat for a few minutes.
3. Add the remaining ingredients through to curry as you stir to ensure it combines well.
4. Add the cauliflower and bring to a boil.
5. Reduce the heat to low, then cover the lid of the pot and let the food simmer until the cauliflower is fork-tender. Ensure you stir occasionally until the soup is ready.
6. Serve while still hot, and enjoy!

Nutritional Facts
Per serving:

Calories	253kCal
Fat	2.9g
Carbs	46.5g
Fiber	15.1g
Sugars	18.9g
Protein	18.1g

Sweet Potato Black Bean Chili

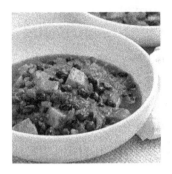

Preparation Time: 30 mins
Servings: 4
Ingredients:

- Extra-virgin oil (1 tbs & 2 tsp)
- One medium-large Sweet potato, peeled and diced
- One large diced onion
- 4 minced garlic cloves
- Chili powder (2 tbs)
- Ground cumin (4 tsp)
- Ground chipotle chili (1/2 tsp)
- Salt (1/4 tsp)
- Water (2 1/2 cups)
- Rinsed black beans (Two 15-ounce cans)
- Diced tomatoes (One 14-ounce can)
- Lime juice (4 tsp)
- Fresh cilantro chopped (1/2 cup)

Directions:
1. Heat the oil in the oven over medium-high heat.
2. Add the sweet potato and onions, cooking as you stir continuously, until the onion begin o soften. This may take about 4 minutes.
3. Add the cumin, garlic, chili powder, chipotle, and salt, and continue to cook for 30 more seconds.
4. Add water and bring to simmer, then cover the lid and reduce the heat to ensure that the food maintains a gentle simmer.
5. Cook until the sweet potato is tender, it'll take about 12 minutes.
6. Add the beans, lime juice and tomatoes, and increase the heat for a while, then reduce the heat to a simmer.
7. Let it cook on simmer for 5 minutes, then remove from heat and stir in the cilantro.

Nutritional Facts
Per Servng:

Calories	307kCal
Fat	8g
Carbs	51g
Protein	12g
Fiber	14g
Sodium	494mg
Potassium	947mg

Broccoli and Cheese Soup

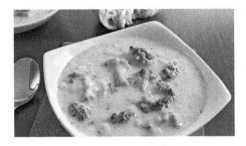

Preparation Time: 30 mins
Servings: 6
Ingredients:

- Cooking spray
- Chopped onion (1 cup)
- Two minced garlic cloves
- Fat-free chicken broth with less sodium (3 cups)
- Broccoli florets (One 16-ounce pack)
- Reduced-fat milk (2 1/2 cups)
- All-purpose flour (1/3 cup)
- Black pepper (1/4 tsp)
- Cubed light processed cheese (8 ounces)

Directions:
1. Coat a large nonstick saucepan with cooking spray and heat it over medium-high heat.
2. Add the garlic, and onion then sauté for 3 minutes until tender.

3. Add the broccoli and the broth and bring the mixture to boil over medium-high heat.

4. Reduce the heat to medium, and continue to cook for 10 minutes.

5. Combine the flour and milk, and stir with a whisk until well blended.

6. Add the milk mixture to the broccoli mixture and let it cook for 5 minutes until slightly thick as you stir constantly.

7. Stir in the pepper and remove the saucepan from the heat. add the cheese and continue to stir until the cheese melts.

8. Place 1/3 of the soup in a food processor or blender, and blend until smooth. Afterwards, return the puree soup mixture to the saucepan.

Nutritional Facts

Per Serving:

Calories	203kCal
Fat	6.3g
Protein	15.6g
Carbs	21.7g
Fiber	2.9g
Cholesterol	24mg
Iron	1.2mg
Sodium	897mg
Calcium	385mg

Cream of Broccoli Soup

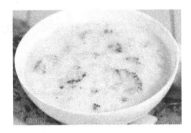

Preparation Time: 40 mins
Servings: 6
Ingredients:

- One onion
- One Celery stalk
- Fresh broccoli (8 cups)
- Homemade Chicken broth (3 cups)
- Nonfat milk (2 cups)
- Cottage cheese (16 ounces)
- Salt to taste

Directions:
1.Chop the celery and onions in a medium size pot, then combine with 3 tablespoons of chicken broth.
2. Heat over medium heat until the onions become tender.
3. Add the fresh broccoli and the remaining chicken broth, then cover and let it simmer for 10 minutes.

4. When the broccoli become tender, blend all the remaining ingredients using an immersion blender.
5. Add the cheese and milk, then simmer the soup for 20 more minutes. This will ensure the soup thickens to the preferable consistency.

Poultry and Meat

Jambalaya

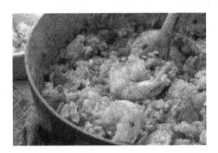

Preparation Time: 1hr 50 mins
Servings: 6
Ingredients:

- One large onion, chopped
- Two diced celery stalks
- One large green bell pepper, cored, seeded, and chopped.
- Two minced garlic cloves(medium sized)
- Diced Boneless, skinless chicken breast (8 ounces)
- Fresh, minced Italian parsley (3tbs)
- One large bay leaf
- Cayenne pepper (1 tsp)
- Tomato sauce (8 ounce can)
- Chicken broth (1 3/4 cups)
- Brown uncooked rice (1 cup)

- Diced, Spicy nitrate-free chicken (4 ounces)
- Sea salt

Directions:

1. Place a wide pot (or a wide, deep skillet) over medium heat. Sauté the bell pepper, onion, garlic, and celery, then cover with lid.
2. Sauté until the onion is translucent.
3. Add the chicken, parsley, cayenne pepper, parsley, and bay leaf into the pot or skillet.
4. Continue to sauté until the chicken no longer looks pink.
5. Stir in the tomato sauce, broth, and rice, then bring to boil.
6. Reduce the heat to low, then cover the lid. Let the food simmer for 1 hour until the rice becomes tender.
7. Season the jambalaya with salt and pepper, then serve sprinkled with the fresh parsley.

Nutritional Facts
Per Serving:

Calories	159.2kCal
Fat	3.1g
Cholesterol	24.1mg
Sodium	893.4mg
Carbs	21.6g
Fiber	3.4g
Protein	12.8g

Meat Loaf with Vegetables

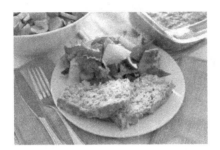

Preparation Time: 1 hr
Servings: 6
Ingredients:

- Extra-virgin olive oil/ vegetable oil (1 tbs)
- 1 chopped onion
- 1/2 Chopped red bell pepper
- 1/2 chopped green bell pepper
- Extra-lean ground beef (1/2 pound)
- Chunky salsa (1 cup)
- 1 beaten egg
- Salt (3/4 tsp)
- Ground black pepper (1/2 tsp)
- 1 Minced garlic clove
- Cooked brown rice (1/2 cup)

Directions:
1. Prepare the rice according to manufacture directions.
2. Preheat the oven to 350 F.
2. In a small skillet, heat the oil over medium heat.
3. Add the onion and bell peppers, then cook for 5 more minutes until the onions become tender.
4. Combine the turkey, beef, turkey, salt, egg, salsa, garlic, and pepper.
5. Place the mixture in a round baking dish.
6. Bake for 45 mins, or until the meat is no longer pink.
7. Serve while still hot and enjoy!

Nutritional Facts
Per Servings:

Calories	225kCal
Fat	10g
Carbs	16g
Protein	17g
Fiber	1g
Sodium	366mg
Cholesterol	79mg

Thai Grilled Beef with String Beef

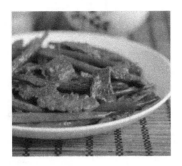

Preparation Time: 30 mins
Servings: 4
Ingredients:

- Flank steak (1 1/2 pound)
- Extra-virgin olive oil, divided (2tsp)
- Ground pepper
- Salt
- Lime juice (1/4 cup)
- Asian fish sauce (1 tbs)
- Minced chili (1 tsp) or chili paste (1/4 tsp)
- Granular sugar substitute (1 tsp)
- Chopped Fresh cilantro (1 cup)
- Thinly sliced scallions (1/2 cups)
- Trimmed string beans (1 pound)

Directions:

1. Heat the grill pan or the grill to high.
2. Rub 1 tsp of oil on each side of the steak, and season with pepper and salt.
3. Grill for about 4 minutes each side until desired doneness.
4. Remove the steak from the heat and set it on a cutting board for 5 minutes.
5. Whisk the chili paste, lime juice, sugar substitute, fish sauce, cilantro, and scallions, in a large mixing bowl.
6. Heat salted water in a saucepan until it boils, then add the beans and cook for 3 minutes until crisp tender, before you drain.
7. Thinly slice the steak, then toss with lime juice mixture. ensure that you also toss in any remaining steak juices from the board.
8. Stir in the beans before you serve.

Nutritional Facts
Per serving:

Calories	340kCal
Fat	17g
Carbs	10g
Protein	38g
Fiber	3g
Sodium	530mg

Roasted Chicken Pomodoro

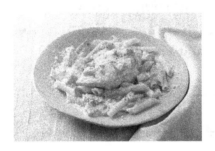

Preparation Time: 20 minutes
Servings: 4
Ingredients:

- Roasted Chicken Tenders
- Water (2 tsp)
- Eggplant, thinly diced
- 2 Tomatoes, thinly sliced
- Canola oil (1 tsp)
- Capers
- Onion (1/2 cup)
- salt and pepper

Directions:

1. Prepare the chicken tenders from frozen state.
2. Remove the container from carton.
3. Cut 1-inch vents on 2 areas of the film
4. Microwave on high for about 2-3 1/2 minutes.
5. Remove the film and stir.

6. Place the contents in a medium saucepan and add the rest of the of the ingredients and cook on medium high heat, until thoroughly cooked.
7. Set the meal aside for a minute or two.
8. Serve and enjoy!

Nutritional Facts
Per serving:

Calories	230kCal
Fat	13g
Fiber	5g
Protein	21g
Cholesterol	55mg

Broccoli and Cheese stuffed chicken breast

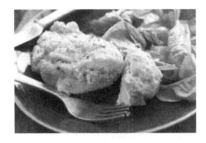

Preparation Time: 50 mins
Servings: 4
Ingredients:

- Chicken breast with rib meat
- Broccoli
- Pasteurized, processed American and Swiss cheese
- Water
- Rice starch
- Vegetable oil
- Enriched Bleached wheat flour
- Lemon juice concentrate
- Rosemary citrus topical
- Roasted chicken
- Salt
- Vinegar
- Sugar
- Soy lecithin

Directions:

1. Prepare the frozen chicken breasts according to product heating instructions.
2. Remove from wrapper, and place in microwave.
3. Microwave on high heat for about 2 1/2 minutes, then set aside for a minute.
4. stuff the chicken with the rest of the ingredients accordingly.
5. Preheat the oven to 350 F.
6. Place the stuffed breasts on baking sheet and bake for 35 minutes until golden brown.

Nutritional Facts
Per Serving:

Calories	210kCal
Fat	10g
Cholesterol	70mg
Sodium	430mg
Carbs	4g
Protein	17g

Spicy Buffalo and Asparagus with Miracle Noodles

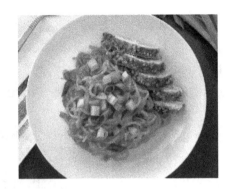

Preparation Time: 40 mins
Servings: 1
Ingredients:

- Buffalo tenderloin (100g)
- Diced onions (1/4 cup)
- Chopped garlic (5tbs)
- Grated fresh ginger (2 tsp)
- Blanketed slivered asparagus (1 cup)
- Chicken broth (1/4 cup)
- Soy sauce (1 tbs)
- Red pepper chili flake (1/4 tbs)
- Toasted sesame seeds (5 tsp)
- Fresh, chopped basil or cilantro (1 tsp)
- Extra virgin oil (1 tsp)
- Angel hair Miracle Noodles (1 7oz bag)

Directions:
1. Prepare a pot of boiling water before you begin to cook.
2. Heat up a 14-inch non-stick sauté pan.
3. Add the virgin oil, then Sauté the meat until it starts browning on both sides.
4. Add in the onions and continue to sauté until softened.
5. Add the ginger and garlic, then stir in the sesame seeds.
6. Add the soy sauce and chicken broth, then bring it up to a high simmer.
7. Prepare the Magic noodles according to the manufacture's description.
8. Sprinkle the noodles with chili flakes and continue to stir.
9. Add the entire mixture to the bowl.
10. Serve hot and enjoy!

Nutritional Facts
Per Serving:

Calories	252.9kCal
Fat	7.6g
Cholesterol	62.3mg
Sodium	1,198.3mg
Carbs	15.1g
Fiber	4.3g
Protein	32.5g

Fish and Seafood

Cajun Shrimp with Steamed Cabbage

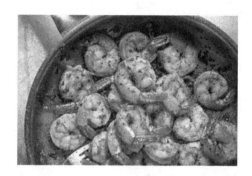

Preparation Time: 1 hr
Servings: 4
Ingredients:

What you'll need for the Creole Seasoning:-

- Paprika (1 tbs)
- Black pepper cracked (1/2 tbs)
- Kosher Salt (1/2 tbs)
- Granulated garlic (1 tsp)
- Dried thyme (1 tsp)
- Dried oregano (1 tsp)
- Dried basil (1 tsp)
- Cayenne (1/4 tsp)

Make sure that you combine all these ingredients ensuring that the seasoning is thoroughly mixed

- Large Shrimp (300g)
- Louisiana Hot sauce, cayenne sauce
- Cabbage leaves (1/2 head or 4 cups)
- Sliced basil (6 fresh leaves)

Directions:
1. Preheat your grill. Place a 2qt pot of water on your grill and bring to boil.
2. Season shrimp with the Creole seasoning and grill until cooked through.
3. Remove from heat and season with Cayenne sauce.
4. Place the cabbage leaves into a pot with salted boiling water, then turn down the heat.
5. Let the cabbage simmer until wilted, then remove and strain the water.
6. Chop the hot cabbage leaves and then season with fresh basil, pepper and salt.
7. Serve, and enjoy!

Nutritional Facts
Per Serving:

Calories	144.9kCal
Fat	2.5g

Cholesterol	168.7mg
Sodium	715.7mg
Carbs	8.6g
Fiber	3.6g
Protein	22.6g

Grilled Shrimp and Raab

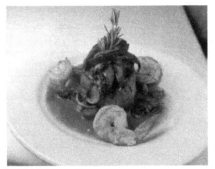

Preparation Time: 30 mins
Servings: 4
Ingredients:

- Shrimp
- 2 bunches of Raab
- Sriracha

Directions:
1. Prepare the shrimp.
2. Preheat Grill.
3. Dip the Raab in salted water then drain.
4. Lay the Raab across the grill and season with salt and pepper, turning when they start to char.
5. Repeat this process on the sides of the shrimps, as you season them.
6. Serve a cup of Raab, with siracha, with 100g of shrimp.

Nutritional Facts

Per Serving:

Calories	181.1kCal
Fat	2.2g
Cholesterol	195.0mg
Sodium	466.4mg
Carbs	8.8g
Fiber	6.1g
Protein	29.3g

Sweet Potato Tuna Patties

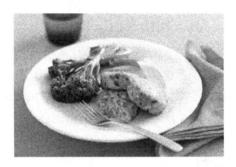

Preparation Time: 35mins
Servings: 3
Ingredients:

- One medium sweet potato
- Minced garlic (1 tsp)
- Chunk light tuna packed in water (2 7oz cans)
- Diced red onions (1 cup)
- Olive Oil (2 tbs)
- Salt
- Pepper

Directions:
1. Peel the sweet potato then slice it into 5 equal portions.
2. Boil the potato in water for approximately 15 minutes, until they become tender.

3. Drain the water, then place the portions into a large bowl, and mash with a fork.

4. Open the canned tuna, drain the excess liquid, and then place the tuna into a bowl along the onions, garlic, pepper, and salt.

5.Combine all the ingredients and form patties.

6. Heat the non-stick pan, the spray the oil.

7. Cook the patties for about 2 minutes on both sides

Nutritional Facts

Per Serving:

Calories	283.7kCal
Fat	13.5g
Cholesterol	50.0mg
Sodium	573.3mg
Carbs	13.3g
Fiber	1.8g
Protein	27.0g

Foil Baked Fish

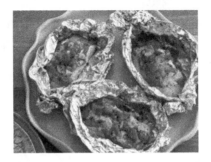

Preparation Time: 50 mins
Serving: 3
Ingredients:

- 4 fish fillets
- Green beans (1 cup)
- Yellow squash (1 cup)
- Dill (1 teaspoon)
- Olive oil (1 tablespoon)
- 1 lime
- Thawed Beans (1/4 cup)

Directions:

1. Brush each fillet with olive oil, then season with pepper and salt.
2. Sprinkle with dill and place on a sheet of aluminum foil.
3. Toss in you cup of squashed beans to the foil and squeeze a bit of lime juice.

4. Repeat the process with each fillet, placing each of them in their own separate foil.

5. Wrap the fish together with the veggies carefully inside the foil and close into a tight packet.

6. Cook the fish on a baking sheet for 15 minutes at 350 F.

Nutritional Facts

Per Serving:

Calories	205.9kCal
Total Fat	4.4 g
Cholesterol	73.3 mg
Sodium	171.4 mg
Potassium	889.3 mg
Carbohydrate	13.4 g
Dietary Fiber	3.9 g
Sugars	6.7 g
Protein	32.4g

Tender Juicy Lemon Baked Cod Recipe

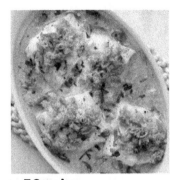

Preparation Time: 50 mins
Servings: 2-3
Ingredients:

- 2 lb cod fillet (any white fish)
- Olive oil (1/4 cup)
- Lemon juice (2 Tbs)
- Gluten free all purpose flour (1/4 cup)
- dash of paprika

Directions:

1. Chop the fillets into serving sizes.
2. In sauce pan or micro-wave, heat olive oil, then add lemon juice to the olive oil.
3. In a different dish, mix together all purpose flour, pepper And salt.
4. Dip the fish into the lemon mix. Ensure that you properly coat on all sides.

5. Dip the lemon-mixed fish into the flour mix. Ensure that you also properly coat on all sides.

6. Place the fillets in an ungreased baking dish, and then sprinkle the entire dish with paprika.

7. Bake the fish uncovered in oven at 350 F for 25-30 minutes.

8. Garnish with lemon wedges and parsley.

9. Serve the fillets. Enjoy!

Nutritional Facts

Per Serving:

Calories	148.8
Total Fat	1.2 g
Cholesterol	77.9 mg
Sodium	110.5 mg
Potassium	345.7 mg
Protein	32.3 g

DESSERTS

Chocolate Cake with Peanut Butter Frosting

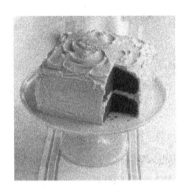

Preparation Time:40 mins

Servings:9

Ingredients:

- Canola oil (1/4 cup)
- 1 large egg
- Vanilla (1 tsp)
- Brown sugar (1/4 cup)
- Splenda Granula (1 cup)
- Low-fat buttermilk (1 cup)
- WW pastry flour (1 1/4 cups)
- Baking soda (1 tsp)
- Dutch-Process cocoa powder (1/4 cup)
- Hot water (1/4 cup)

Directions:

1. Preheat the oven to 350, then spray your baking pan(preferably 8x8-inch) with non-sticking cooking spray.
2. Whisk the egg in the oil in a large bowl for 1 minute till the mixture is frothy & thick.
3. Add in the sugar, vanilla, and splenda then continue to mix for 2 more minutes, until smooth and thick. After preparing the mixture thoroughly, add the buttermilk.
4. Mix the baking powder, flour, baking soda, and cocoa powder thoroughly in a bowl, before adding them to your liquid mixture.
5. Whisk properly for about 2 minutes until the batter is nice and smooth, then pour the hot water into the batter, mixing once more until nice and smooth(the batter will be thin).
6. Pour the batter onto the cake pan, and ensure that all the air bubbles are removed by tapping the pan.
7. Bake for approximately 20 minutes (depending on the equipment it can sometimes take about 30-35 mins), until the center springs back when touched. You can use a cake tester.
8. Remove the cake from the oven and let it cool before you serve.

Nutritional Facts
Per serving:

Calories	160kCal
Carb	22g
Sugar	8g
Protein	3g
Fat	7g
Sat	1g
Fiber	1g
Sodium	200mg

Jeremy's Apple Puree

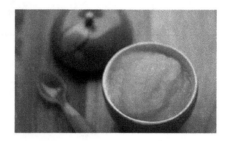

Preparation Time: 10 mins
Servings: 1
Ingredients:

- One medium Apple
- Ground cinnamon (1 tbsp)
- Water (1/4 cup)
- Vanilla Cream Stevia (12 drops)

Directions:
1. Combine all the ingredients in a food processor, and pulse until smooth.
2. Pour into bowl and microwave on high for 3 minutes.

Nutritional Facts
Per Serving:

Calories	112.7kCal
Fat	0.5g
Sodium	3.8mg

Carbs	30.5g
Fiber	8.1g
Protein	0.8g

Jeremy's Cocoa Delight- Cocoa Crack

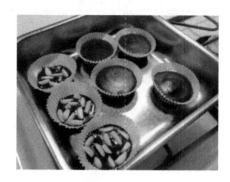

Preparation Time: 5 mins
Servings: 1
Ingredients:

- Coconut Oil (3 tbsp)
- Unsweetened Cocoa Powder (3 tbsp)
- Stevia or liquid (3 packets)

Directions:
1. Mix all the ingredients and microwave until the coconut oil liquefies.
2. Stir the ingredients until there's no presence of lumps.
3. Pour onto wax paper then place it in the freezer for approximately 20 mins.
4. Before freezing, you can add some crushed nuts, or almonds if you so desire. In addition to that, the

various flavors of the liquid stevia will add some nice tastes.

Nutritional Facts
Per Serving:

Calories	388.8kCal
Fat	43.0g
Sodium	3.4mg
Carbs	8.8g
Fiber	5.4g
Protein	3.2g

Chocolate Cream Cheese Cupcakes

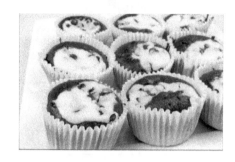

Preparation Time: 15 mins
Servings: 12
Ingredients:
For preparing the cupcake mix: -

- Coconut Flour (1/3 cup)
- Unsweetened Cocoa (1/3 cup)
- Coconut Oil (1/3 cup)
- Salt (1/3 tsp)
- Baking Soda (1/2 tsp)
- Truvia (1/4 cup)
- Pure Vanilla Extract (1 tsp)
- Four Whole large eggs

For preparing the filling mix: -

- Cream cheese (1 3 oz pack)

- Truvia (6 packs)
- Sugar free chocolate chips (1/4 cups)

Directions:

1. Pre-heat your oven to 375F.
2. Mix the chocolate chips, cream cheese and truvia together, then put it aside.
3. Mix the rest of the ingredients together, then place them in equal proportions inside the cupcake papers.
4. Make a hole 1/2 size of cupcake in the center to bottom after wetting your finger with water.
5. When you've completed this, fill each hole with the cream cheese filling.
6. Bake for 7 minutes, then cover with a towel and let the cupcakes cool.

Nutritional Facts
Per serving:

Calories	121.4kCal
Fat	10.8g
Cholesterol	7.7mg
Sodium	156.2mg
Carbs	10.5g
Protein	2.8g

Carrot-Pineapple Muffins

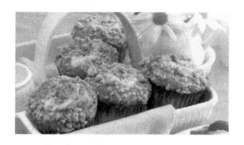

Preparation Time: 30 mins
Serving: 18
Ingredients:

- Crushed pineapple in juice (8 ounces)
- All-purpose flour (1 cup)
- Whole wheat flour (1 cup)
- Brown packed sugar (1/2 cup)
- Baking powder (1 tbs)
- Baking soda (1/2 tsp)
- Salt (1/4 tsp)
- Skim milk (1 cup)
- Egg substitute (1/2 cup)
- Unsweetened applesauce (1/4 cup)
- Vegetable oil (2 tbs)
- Finely shredded carrot (1 cup)
- Golden raisins (1/2 cup)

Directions:

1. Preheat the oven to 400 F.
2. Drain the pineapple, reserving the juice for another use.
3. Press the pineapple between the paper towels to remove the excess moisture, then set it aside.
4. In a medium bowl, combine the flours as well as the next 4 ingredients, then make a hole in the center of the mixture.
5. Mix the milk as well the next three ingredients, before adding the mix to the dry ingredients. Continue to stir until moist.
6. Stir in the carrot, pineapple, and raisins, then divide the batter evenly among the muffin cups after coating the cups with cooking spray.
7. Bake the muffins for 20 minutes until they turn golden.
8. Remove them from the oven immediately.

Nutritional Facts
Per Serving:

Calories	126kCal
Fat	3g
Protein 3g	
Carbs	24g
Sodium	172mg

CONCLUSION

If you're looking around for a new diet to try, chances are you've come across tons of different diet plans, and maybe you're feeling a little overwhelmed or confused. That's natural: From low-carb to zero sugar to paleo, the options seem endless. Despite what you see on the Internet, no single diet works for everyone. Rather, you'll have to experiment with different ways of eating to find out what works best for you.

The South Beach Diet may be a good place to start if you're interested in a quick reboot to help you feel better and get rid of bloat, but you shouldn't remain in the first phase of this diet for long. Instead, prioritize eating whole, nutrient-dense foods, and foods that make you feel good. Additionally, you would benefit from talking with a doctor or dietitian before beginning any weight-loss program or diet.

Part 2

Introduction

The following chapters will discuss some of the basics that you should know if you would like to get started with the South Beach Diet. Many people who have gone on this diet plan have gone on other ones in the past and find that none of them work as they promise. They want something that will work, something they can stick with for the long time, and maybe something that is a bit drastic to help them lose the weight. For some, the South Beach Diet may seem a little strict, but it is meant to train the body to know what foods are good and which ones are bad in a safe and wholesome way.

In this guidebook, we are going to spend some time talking about the South Beach Diet and what it all entails. We will talk about the foods that you are allowed to eat during the different phases (this diet plan is composed of three different phases, two of which to work with losing weight and the last one to help you maintain that weight loss) and any other information that you need during these stages. We will also provide you with 40 recipes, split up into the 3 different phases, that will help you to stick through this during any phase you are in while still eating delicious foods.

When you are tired of other diet plans just not working for you and you want to finally see some of the success that you have been working so hard for, make sure to check out this guidebook and learn everything that you need about the South Beach Diet and all the great recipes that go with it!

There are plenty of books on this subject on the market, thanks again for choosing this one! Every effort was made to ensure it is full of as much useful information as possible, please enjoy!

Chapter 1: What is the South Beach Diet?

There are many different types of diets that you are able to go on during your life. Many of them are going to promise to help you lose weight and feel great, but most of them will leave you feeling like you failed in some way. Some are gong to be too restrictive and make you just drink juices or something else that is equally unhealthy all of the time. Others are going to make you concentrate on eating the wrong kinds of foods and then you will just see weight gain or other issues. None of them are going to work like you will find in the South Beach Diet.

This diet is one that is meant to help you to stay safe while losing weight quickly. While there are some diets out there that encourage you to skip meals and not eat enough calories, all three of the phases on this diet plan, even Phase 1 that is seen as the most restrictive and hardest to follow, will allow you to eat three meals each day and they all include two snacks as well. Your only requirement is to cut out the certain foods in each section and to eat until you feel pleasantly full. You won't have to skip out on snacks or meals unless you are too hungry for them.

The portions of food that you eat (and this is real and good food), will help you to get all the nutrients that you need. You will get high fiber carbs in the form of unsaturated fats, protein sources that are lean, dairy that is low fat, vegetables, whole grains, and fruits that are so good for you. Even in the first phase, you are allowed to have a little dessert to make things easier, as long as you make the right choices with this. After finishing your first two weeks on this diet plan, you will be able to even add on some red wine on occasion to the diet plan.

The goals that the South Beach Diet has include helping you to not only lose the weight in a safe and effective manner, but to help you stay fit and healthy for the rest of your life. this is not something that you can do if you go around feeling starved or tired all the time or when you are eating all the wrong foods that just add on more weight.

Yes, there are some critics to this diet who think it is too restrictive for you to follow, but there has to be some changes in the way that you eat if you would like to see changes in your weight. Too many times we take it easy on ourselves when it comes to picking out the diet plan or the foods we can eat, and this is why the weight is still there. We need to have the first phase of this diet plan, and even some of the restrictiveness of the second phase, to help us to understand the good foods we are allowed to eat so that when we do indulge, we don't go too overboard.

Now, there are three distinct phases of the South Beach Diet. The first two are meant to help with the weight loss part and the third phase is more of a maintenance to happen after you have lost all of the weight. All of these are going to work together to help you to become fit and healthy and you are able to go back to any of the phases that you would like if you start to see a backwards trend in your weight again. Keep in mind that all of these also have different rules for the kinds of foods that you are allowed to consume on them so be careful with this part. Let's take a look these different phases so we have a better understanding of how you would work with each one.

Phase 1:

When you are ready to begin on this particular diet plan, you are going to enter into Phase 1. This is the shortest phase out of all of them, but it is also one of the most restrictive in terms of what you are allowed to eat. Luckily, this one is going to be for only 2 weeks, but it is meant to help stop the cravings and to really teach the body what it is allowed to have and not have. Those who go on the South Beach Diet with a lot of weight to lose will notice that they will have a lot of cravings for refined starches and sugary foods during this part, but you will just need to hold off on those during this time.

This phase is helping you to not only get a great start with losing some of that weight, but it makes the levels of sugars in the blood more stable so that you can minimize your cravings later on. You are going to spend your time eating healthy and lean protein, such as turkey, chicken, shellfish, and fish, lots of vegetables, and nuts, low fat dairy, eggs, good fats, and so on.

During this phase, you will not feel deprived other than the cravings that may sneak up, but these are not harmful to your health. You are allowed to have three meals each day along with two snacks, and it is fine to have a dessert. But you will not be able to eat any sugars (even the sugars that are found inside of fruits) nor will you be allowed to eat any starches such as rice, pasta, and bread.

This stage is going to seem really hard at first. Your body is going to have a lot of cravings as you get rid of all those starches and sugars out of the body, and it will seem impossible. But if you are planning out your meals correctly, you should not feel hungry at all until it is time to get for another meal. If it gets hard, just remember that the first phase is only going to last for two weeks and then you are allowed to add quite a few of these foods back into the diet.

Another thing that you should remember, in addition to which foods you are allowed to eat and which ones you should avoid, is that exercise is important to this phase as well as the other phases. It is going to improve a lot of different parts of your health and will make it easier to see some of the results that you want.

During Phase 1, you are going to see that the weight loss is happening pretty rapidly, which gives a lot of positive reinforcement for this diet plan and can help you to stick with it if you can get over the cravings. When you are done, you will have gotten rid of some of the cravings and can even stabilize your blood sugars a bit better. This will make it easier when you go into the second phase because you will be better able to control the foods that you eat when some of them are reintroduced into the diet.

Phase 2:

In some cases, you will be able to get started right out with Phase 2 when you go on the South Beach Diet. If you are only trying to lose 10 pounds or less on this diet, you aren't someone who has to deal with cravings all the time, or you are just doing this as a way to improve your health, you can skip right to phase 2. For those who started with Phase 1 and then moved into Phase2, you are going to notice that you will keep going with a steady weight loss, but it will slow down. You should also notice that a lot of the cravings that you had in the past will subside.

This is the phase where you will be able to add in a lot more of the foods that were taken away during Phase 1 since now you are able to control the cravings a bit better than before. Some of the foods that you are able to include in the diet now that you are in Phase 2 include good carbs such as whole fruits, whole wheat pasta and breads, and some of the root vegetables. On some occasions, you will be able to add in a glass of white or red wine to your meal.

Remember that the weight loss is going to be slower during this period because the diet is not as restrictive at this point. This can sometimes be discouraging to people who were excited about the quick weight loss they were going through. The goal here is to get to a healthy weight that you are able to maintain with your good eating and lifestyle habits for the long term and losing weight quickly isn't something that any of us are able to handle for too long.

This is the phase that is going to help you to stay on the diet rather than see it as a quick fix. You are going to stay within phase 2 until you reach your goal weight or the weight that you are happy with. This means that the length of time that you spend in this phase is going to vary between people. Some just have a few pounds to lose and will be able to get out of this one quickly and others could spend months here working to get the weight off. Go at the pace that is right for you and keep in mind that it does take a lot longer for those who have more weight to lose.

If you do feel that you are hitting a plateau in this stage and you still have quite a bit of weight to lose, consider going back to phase 1 for a week or two to help get it kick started again.

Phase 3:

And finally you are going to get into Phase 3. This is the one that you are going to enter when you finally reach the healthy weight for you. The guidelines that are in Phase 3 are the same that other healthy Americans should follow, even those who have never had to deal with their weight. If you followed the other two phases of this diet the right way, you should now know how to make some good choices when it comes to the meals that you can consume and you will be able to take choices from any of the food groups and still stay healthy.

During this phase, you are allowed to eat from any food group, but you still need to behave and not go overboard. Sure you can have a cookie or something sweet, but stick with one and keep the rest of the meals as healthy as possible to avoid issues with gaining the weight back. If you dedicated your time to learning how to do the South Beach Diet right, you should be able to have these little cheats without having to worry about losing out the whole way.

Remember that during this process, you are allowed to go back through the phases if you would like at any time. If you are on Phase 3 for some time and feel like your eating habits are getting out of hand again or you have a big event that you would like to lose a few more pounds for, it is possible to spend some time back in Phase 1 or Phase 2 again to help out. While you should be able to stay with Phase 3 for the rest of your life and not gain weight if you do it right, there are always times when life gets in the way and the pounds may sneak back on again. Rather than letting it get out of hand, you can just re-enter a Phase of this diet from before and get things back on track.

The South Beach Diet is meant to help you learn how to work with your body and eat the foods that are good for you. It isn't going to tell you that one food is bad and one is good, but it is going to teach you that some of the foods that you are consuming on a daily basis, especially when you eat them in high amounts, are the reason that you are feeling hungry all the time while gaining weight. When you go through the phases of the South Beach Diet, you take away all of these bad foods that are causing the weight gain and then slowly add them back in so that you learn what is allowed in the body and what you are able to handle. You should be able to make good decisions for your health by the time you get to the third phase so that you can keep the weight off, even if you have a little cheat on occasion.

Chapter 2: The Truth About Carbs in the Body

When it comes to most of the diet plans that you have tried in the past, there is one thing that most of them will have in common. Most of these are going to tell you that fat is the enemy, that these fats are the things that are making you sick and making it hard to lose weight. If you are able to reduce the amount of fats that you are eating, you will be able to lose weight.

There are a number of problems with this though. The first issue is that these diets see that there are differences between bad fats and good fats. There is a difference when it comes to the type of fats that you eat. If you are eating saturated fats from your favorite fast food restaurant each day, you are going to get sick and have all the issues that those other diet plans promise. But there are plenty of healthy fats that you can consume, ones that come in healthy protein sources and fish that will fuel the body, help the mind, and just make you feel better overall. If you miss out on some of these healthy fats, you are going to end up causing a lot of harm to the body because it is missing out on some important nutrients that it needs.

The next issue is what you are replacing these fats with. Since you aren't getting your nutrition from the healthy fats that the body needs, you are going to need to get them from somewhere. Most of these diets ask you to get the nutrition from carbs. But just like with fats, there are good carbs and bad carbs and these are not distinguished from in these diet plans either.

When you consume carbs, especially since most people are going to choose the bad carbs instead of the good ones, you are consuming a really unhealthy form of energy. Your body is not going to be able to process this properly, which is why you feel that burst of energy in the beginning and then go through a big crash shortly after. This is because the carbs that you are consuming are being converted into sugars inside the body, sugars that you aren't using up as quickly as you should and which can make you feel sick, worn down, and add to belly fat in no time.

These diets have been telling it to you wrong for so long now. You are eating the wrong kind of nutrition into your diet each day, taking in the harmful carbs that are adding to excess fat around the body and raising your blood sugars to abnormal heights. You need those good fats in your life if you would like to be healthy, but too many times we are told that all fats are bad, so we learn how to stay away from them.

Fats are better for the body. They are the most efficient form of energy for the body possible. When you bring these into the body, you are not converting them into something that is hard on the body (such as carbs that will turn into sugars and not be used). You are bringing in something that will provide you with energy all day long. Some people do notice a lag in their energy levels right at the beginning, but this is mostly because the body is looking for carbs and it takes it a bit to learn to rely on the fat stores instead.

But there are going to be some pretty amazing things that happen when you start to reduce the amount of carbs that you are consuming in favor of more fats. First, you are going to have more energy because the fat is able to keep the body going for a much longer time. The body is going to see the fat that you are consuming and just eat it up, helping you to feel ready to take on the day. And then, when the body is done using the fat that you consume, it is going to turn around and start eating up the fat that is stored all around your body. Once the body starts to use fats instead of carbs as the main source of energy, you will be able to see it eat through the body fat without any extra work!

Another benefit is that foods that are full of the healthy fats are the ones that will fill you up for much longer. Think back to those diets that you were on in the past; where there many days that you just felt hungry all the time, no matter how many calories you took in? This is most likely because you aren't taking in any of the fats that you need, the ones that fill you up and make you feel full and satisfied after a meal.

While on the South Beach Diet, you are going to learn to control the amount of carbs that you are eating, especially during the first two phases. This diet doesn't assume that all carbs are bad (there are plenty of carbs that can be good and provide good nutrition), but it recognizes that most of us don't know how to determine good carbs from bad and most of us eat way too much of them. We need to learn how to monitor the carbs that we are eating and so we take most of them away, and focus instead on some of the healthy fats and other foods that we are allowed to eat on this diet plan.

There are still plenty of great meals that you will be able to enjoy when you are on this kind of diet plan, but you will have to shift the focus that you are eating with in order to see the best results. The good news is that these high fat meals are going to taste good and be filling, so you will eat fewer calories, without feeling deprived, and still be able to lose weight all at the same time.

The South Beach Diet is the perfect way to help you to work with the carbs that are in your body. On your typical American diet, you are spending a lot of time consuming the carbs that you just don't need. You are taking in large amounts of baked goods, pizzas, breads, and other things. And when the cravings come around, it is hard to say no and just stay away from them. But the South Beach Diet is going to help.

It is important to realize that the South Beach Diet is not against carbs. This diet plan realizes that there is some importance to the carbs in your diet, but it is trying to help you to learn what carbs are good and in what amounts you should be eating those carbs. Yes, the first phase of the diet is going to pretty much eliminate the carbs as much as possible, but this is not because all carbs are bad; it is simply a way to help you quickly get through the issues you have with cravings. Once you get past that first two-week period, you can slowly add in those carbs and when you get to the third phase, you can eat any carbs that you would like as long as you do so in moderation and you are careful to eat the ones that are whole wheat or whole grain.

While this diet plan is going to seem hard in the beginning, especially when those cravings start to come and bug you, you will find that it is the fastest and safest way to get rid of those cravings so that you can make informed and healthy choices about the carbs that you consume. Most of this diet is going to focus on the healthy produce and the healthy fats that you can consume, but if you learn how to get rid of the cravings and instead go for the good carbs that are going to fill you up (mainly whole wheat and plenty of produce), you are allowed to have some carbs on this diet plan.

So what are you going to eat when you are on the South Beach Diet? We just talked about how you will need to limit your carb intake on the first two phases of this diet, but what is there left to eat. When you are on the first phase, you are going to concentrate on healthy fats and proteins, such as lean turkey and chicken and lots of fish. You can have a few vegetables, but you will concentrate more on the low fat dairy, the protein, and the healthy oils.

Then on the second phase, you are able to add in more of the carbs if you would like. This is going to include healthy carbs though and you will want to go pretty slowly to get started. For example, maybe start the first week with an extra serving of vegetables and then move in to having some fruits in there and finally get to adding in the carbs, once you know that your carvings are better under control.

The second phase can last some time depending on how much weight you are trying to lose, but when you get to the third phase, you will be able to enjoy any of the carbs you would like, as long as you are taking them in moderation. This means you can have that snack or dessert on occasion, you just need to be smart about it. By this point you should know more about your body and what it is allowed to have and how to avoid the cravings so indulging on occasion is not going to be such a bad thing.

While the other diets are going to keep telling you that the fats are bad and the carbs are good, you will see that they just don't have the success that you are used to when working with this great diet plan.

Chapter 3: The 3 Phases in South Beach Diet and Foods Allowed in Each One

There are three phases that are recognized on the South Beach Diet. Each of these are meant to help you to lose weight and learn how to properly eat different foods in your life. The first phase is going to be the most restrictive when it comes to the foods that are allowed, but you will find that all of the phases have some rules about food so that you learn how to properly eat for weight loss and weight loss maintenance.

The Phase 1 Foods

The first phase is one of the most important parts of the South Beach Diet, even though it is only going to last for two weeks. This phase is going to help you to go from your old habits to healthier ones that are allowed on this diet plan. Most Americans are used to taking in a lot of unhealthy carbs ad foods and eating way too much of them. This means that they are going to take on foods that are making them gain weight and not feel good. During the first phase, we are going to eliminate a lot of the foods that are causing the weight gain and the bad cravings so that we can break the cycle and learn how to eat in a much healthier way.

The first phase is one of the hardest ones. This is the diet plan that is trying to make sure that you get rid of some of the cravings that are driving you insane and making it hard to give up your foods. But these cravings are going to be hard to fight so you need to be ready to give them up. You are only going to be allowed a few carbs (like half a cup of vegetables a day) in this phase in order to finally break up the amount of cravings that you are dealing with on a daily basis.

So on this part of the diet, you will be limiting a lot of the foods that you are allowed to eat. But the important part to remember here is that it is for your good health. This phase is hard, but it only lasts you for two weeks before moving on to the second phase and then you are allowed to bring a lot of these carbs back in the second phase after the cravings.

First, let's talk about the meats that you are allowed to eat on the first phase. There are many great meat sources that you are allowed to eat, you just need to make sure that you are not eating the ones that have been processed and can make you feel really sick with all the sugars and carbs that are added in. Some of the meat options that you are able to enjoy include turkey and Canadian bacon, chicken breast, turkey, lean cuts of beef, boiled ham, lunch meats that are lower in fat, seafood of all kinds, and even soy based meat substitutes.

If you are not a fan of meat or you are a vegetarian, you are able to use many types of beans to ensure that you are able to find the right amount of protein to make you feel good. Some of the most popular forms of beans that you are allowed to eat on this diet include pinto beans, chickpeas, great northern beans, and black eyed peas.

Nuts are another part of the South Beach Diet that you are allowed to consume and enjoy. You will need to limit the serving to just one each day. This is enough to allow you to get all the good nutrients that you need out of the nuts, but still makes sure that you don't take in too many that will make you feel overwhelmed with too much fat.

There are some limits on the types of vegetables that you are allowed to consume. Most of them are going to be fine, but there are a lot that have more carbs in them than you are allowed on this part of the diet. You will be able to add them back in later on but this phase is going to restrict them a little bit. Remember that since you are restricting your carbs on this part that you are only allowed to have about half a cup of these to stay healthy and to beat the cravings. Some of the vegetables that you can have on this part of the diet plan include peppers, Brussels Sprouts, Broccoli, Cauliflower, okra, spinach, sprouts, lettuce, mushrooms, onions, squash, and tomatoes.

In addition, you are allowed to have some dairy and fats in order to stay full and happy on this part of the diet plan. It is common to eat cheeses that are low in fat, salad dressing that is low in sugar (and only a few tablespoons of this each day), avocado, a few tablespoons of a healthy oil, egg whites and whole eggs, and cottage cheese.

You may notice on this section that you are not allowed to have any fruits. These are high in carbs and are not the healthiest option. Most fruits are considered healthy of course, but while you are going through this part of the diet and working to get through the cravings that are making you unhealthy, you will need to refrain from eating fruits for now. The good news is that you will be able to add them back in later on.

These are the major food groups that you need to focus on when you are trying to get started on the South Beach Diet. It is restrictive, but you are going to notice that your cravings get smaller and smaller as you go through the two weeks and you will notice that you can lose a good amount of weight on this phase of the diet plan too, making it easier to find enough encouragement to keep on going through these two weeks.

The Phase 2 Foods

After you get done with the first phase of the South Beach Diet (thank goodness after all that hard work and missing out on some of your favorite foods!) it is time to move on to the second phase. This one is still going to have some restrictions, but it is also going to help allow a few more things back on. You will be able to have some fruits again for example. But remember that you still need to be a bit limiting on what you are allowed to consume so that you are still able to lose the weight during this time.

During this phase, you will be allowed to eat the same foods as the first phase, but you can also start to reintroduce some more foods to the diet. You should go slowly though. It is not a good idea to flood the body with carbs, even good carbs that are found inside of fruits and vegetables, because this is going to trigger the cravings to come back and can make it so you need to re-enter phase 1 again. You should slowly add in some healthy carbs to the diet, but do it slowly and a little bit at a time.

You may feel that adding in a serving a day for a week may be a good idea. Then you can get a few more that you were supposed to be avoiding, but you still aren't overdoing it either. Perhaps start out by adding in some more fruits and vegetables to start for a few weeks, such as for treats so that your body gets used to the healthy carbs first. Once you are done with this part, you can start to add in some of the other carbs, such as whole grain pastas and whole grain breads, as long as you go slowly and add them in without flooding the system.

During this phase, you will also want to be careful with not taking in too much bread. This is the phase where you are allowed to eat some products that are whole grain and some brown rice, but you do need to be careful. There is a lot of marketing that promises the product is how you want, but when you look at the ingredients, you will find that this is false. You should always check the label and make sure that it has at least 3g or more of fiber in each serving and that it has not been processed.

In addition, you are allowed to add in some alcohol, as long as you do this in moderation. You are not allowed to go out and party each night and say it is part of the South Beach Diet. But if you have a glass of wine with supper, you are able to get some heart benefits with your meal. But taking in more than this can cause more harm than good, especially with all the carbs that you are taking in, and you don't want this.

This is a phase where you should take some time to equip the kitchen in order to get it ready for some healthy living for the rest of your life. Remember that the South Beach Diet is all about finding healthy ways to keep on it for the rest of your life. This is not a fad diet that you go on for a few months and then give up. There are two weight loss phases and then one that is meant to help you to maintain that weight loss for years to come. But one of the steps for you to do this is to make sure that your kitchen is ready to help.

A good place to start is with a scale. This helps you to measure out how much of each food you are consuming so you don't go overboard with the carbs. For example, fruits are really easy to overeat so having a scale around to help you measure it all out can help. Measuring cups, approved food lists, and even making sure to clean out the pantry and only have good foods around can all help you to succeed.

And finally, learning how to eat with mindfulness is important when it comes to being healthy. Most of us overeat because we spend time in front of the television eating, we eat in the car, we scarf down the meal without thinking and so much else. We eat because we are bored or sad or because it is convenient, not because we are hungry.

On the South Beach Diet, you don't need to count the calories as much, but you do need to practice mindful eating. You need to eat when the body is hungry, rather than when you are bored or sad. You need to sit down and enjoy your meals, rather than hurrying through them and eating as much as possible. Taking slow and deliberate bites, prolonging the meal, and just enjoying yourself can really help to make it easier to eat the right amount, while still feeling full, on this diet plan.

During Phase 2, you are still working on losing the weight and feeling good, but you will see that there are still some restrictions on what you are allowed to eat. In addition, the weight loss is going to slow way down. You may lose five to ten pounds in the first few weeks on the South Beach Diet because of all the foods that you are getting rid of and the fact that the body is taking in fewer calories. But things kind of even out on the second phase and you are more likely to lose between 1 and 2 pounds a week instead. You will stick with this phase until you reach your weight loss goals, with perhaps a quick visit back to Phase 1 if you get stuck or need some extra help.

The Phase 3 Foods

When you get to Phase 3, you should be able to add in most of the foods that you had to take out before. This makes it easier for you to eat more of a variety in your diet without being as restrictive as you had to be in some of the other options. You will still need to be careful in this one though. You need to remember that while you are allowed to have a few cheats here and there because you should know how to eat properly for your body by this point, that it can be easy to fall back into old habits and take more calories than you want.

If you stick with what you learned in the South Beach Diet and don't go overboard, you are able to add in all the foods back to your diet. You can have a cheat day with a cookie or another sweet, as long as you keep it in moderation. You should concentrate your efforts on eating healthy and whole foods like fruits, lean meats, whole grains, vegetables, nuts, and dairy that is low in fat and seeds instead of the bad stuff though, even on this part of the diet. You most likely won't be losing weight on this section though since this is more of the maintenance phase of the diet instead of the weight loss part, but you still need to continue to eat the good foods that your body needs to stay healthy.

When it comes to the different phases that are needed in this diet plan, you need to make sure that you are eating the right kinds of foods. Each of these phases is important to help you to really lose the weight and feel good. The different phases are important because they all help you in different ways on this journey to help you to lose weight and feel good.

Chapter 4: Recipes During Phase 1 of the South Beach Diet

Vegetable Hash

Ingredients:

Minced garlic clove (1)
Diced zucchini (2)
Chopped mushrooms (4)
Diced red bell pepper (1)
Salt
Paprika
Thyme
Chopped onion (1)
Olive oil (1 Tbsp.)

Directions:

1.   Bring out a skillet and heat some oil on it. When this is warm, add the thyme, onion, and paprika.
2.   Reduce the heat a bit and then stir this for 7 minutes so the onion can become soft.
3.   Now add in the garlic, zucchini, mushrooms, bell pepper, and salt. Cover the skillet and let it stir for another 4 minutes.
4.   Take off the heat and serve.

Quiche Cups

Ingredients:

Diced onion (1/4 c.)
Green bell pepper (1/4 c.)
Hot pepper sauce (3 drops)
Egg substitute (3/4 c.)
Cheddar cheese (3/4 c.)
Chopped spinach (1 pkg.)

Directions:

1.   Turn on the oven to preheat to 350 degrees. Take out a muffin pan and spray with some cooking spray.
2.   Place the spinach into a container and cook for 2 ½ minutes. Drain out any liquid that is extra.
3.   Bring out a big bowl and combine together the pepper sauce, onion, bell pepper, egg substitute, cheese, and spinach.
4.   Mix this well and divide the mixture between the muffin cups. Place into the oven and let it cook for 20 minutes.

Green Gazpacho

Ingredients:

Olive oil (1 Tbsp.)
Water (2 Tbsp.)
Cayenne (1/8 tsp.)
Lime juice (2 Tbsp.)
Peeled garlic clove (1)
Chopped scallions (2)
Chopped green bell pepper (1)
Chopped lettuce, red leaf (2 c.)
Chopped cucumber (2 ½ lbs.)
Diced avocado (1)
Salt (1/4 tsp.)

Directions:

1.   Take out a blender and puree the cumin, salt, oil, water, lime juice, garlic, scallions, pepper, lettuce, and cucumbers. Season with some more salt if needed.
2.   Move this to a big bowl. Let this chill for a minimum of 2 hours, but overnight is better.
3.   When it is time to serve, peel and dice up the avocado and divide this between 4 bowls before adding the avocado and serving.

Tomato Soup

Ingredients:

White mushrooms (5 oz.)
Red pepper flakes (1/4 tsp.)
Basil (1/4 tsp.)
Oregano (1/4 tsp.)
Minced garlic cloves (4)
Minced celery stalks (2)
Minced onion (1)
Olive oil (1 Tbsp.)
Water (3/4 c.)
Tomato sauce (1 can)
Lima beans (1 can)
Diced tomatoes (1 can)
Diced summer squash (1)

Directions:

1.   Bring out a pan and heat some oil on it. Add the pepper flakes, oregano, basil, garlic, celery, and onion.
2.   Cook this for 5 minutes. Add in the mushrooms and squash. Let these bake a bit longer.
3.   Add in the tomatoes and their juices along with the diced tomatoes and beans. Bring this to a simmer.
4.   Continue to cook until everything is heated through and then serve.

White Bean Soup

Ingredients:

Northern beans (1 can)
Salt
Thyme
Rosemary (1/2 tsp.)
Garlic cloves (2)
Basil (1/2 tsp.)
Chopped celery stalk (1)
Chopped onion (1)
Olive oil (1)
Vegetable broth (1 ½ c.)

Directions:

1.   Bring out a pan and heat it up with the oil inside. Add the salt, thyme, rosemary, basil, garlic, celery, and onion. Let the heat come down a bit and cook a little longer.
2.   When the vegetables are soft, add in the beans and stir. After this is warm, move ¾ of the mixture to a blender and add the broth.
3.   Puree this until smooth and then return to the pan. Bring this to a simmer to make warm and then season with some pepper and salt to taste.

Labne Balls

Ingredients:

Olive oil
Italian seasoning (2 Tbsp.)
Salt (1 tsp.)
Greek yogurt (3 containers)

Directions:

1.   Take out a strainer and line it with a cheesecloth. Place this over a bowl. Bring out a second bowl and combine the salt and yogurt.
2.   Spoon this all into the strainer and then cover with the plastic wrap. Let this set in the fridge for 48 hours. You will notice that you have 1 ½ cups of drained yogurt after this time.
3.   Place the Italian seasonings in a dish. Take out a piece of waxed paper and then roll out the yogurt into small balls. Roll these through the Italian seasonings.
4.   Serve these right away.

Skillet Cod

Ingredients:

Cod fillets (4)
Peguillo peppers (2)
Drained diced tomatoes (1 can)
Pepper
Salt
Minced garlic cloves (3)
Sliced onion (1)
Sliced zucchini (1)
Olive oil (1 Tbsp.)
Parsley (2 Tbsp.)

Directions:

1.   Take out a big skillet and heat some oil. Add the pepper, salt, garlic, onion, and zucchini, letting it cook for 10 minutes.
2.   Now add in the peppers and tomatoes and let it heat for 10 more minutes.
3.   Add the fish into the sauce, making sure to add some to the top. Cover this and let the fish cook until it is opaque, which will take around 10 minutes.
4.   Sprinkle on a bit of parsley and then serve warm.

Tomato and Spinach Salmon

Ingredients:

Baby spinach (3 c.)
Chopped tomatoes (1 lb.)
Minced garlic cloves (2)
Chopped onion (1)
Olive oil (1 Tbsp.)
Pepper
Salt
Salmon fillets (4)
Lemon wedges (4)
Drained capers (1 Tbsp.)

Directions:

1.   Heat up the oven to be at broil. Use some cooking spray to prepare a baking dish.
2.   Place the salmon into the baking dish and season with pepper and salt. Add this to the baking dish.
3.   Broil the salmon for 10 minutes to cook through, but don't turn it.
4.   While the salmon is broiling, bring out your skillet and let the oil cook inside a bit. Add in the onion and garlic, stirring a few times for 7 minutes. Then add in the capers, spinach, and tomatoes and cook another 2 minutes.

5.   Remove the salmon from the oven and put it on 4 plates. Spoon the tomato mixture on top and squeeze a bit of lemon over it. Serve warm.

Pecan Trout

Ingredients:

Olive oil (2 tsp.)
Beaten egg (1)
Salt (1/4 tsp.)
Whole trout (4)
Cayenne (1/8 tsp.)
Garlic clove (1)
Rosemary (1 tsp.)
Pecans (1/2 c.)

Directions:

1.   Heat the oven up to 400 degrees. Lay out a baking sheet and cover it with parchment paper.
2.   Place the cayenne, garlic, rosemary, and pecans into the food processor and chop them until they are fine. Move this to a shallow dish.
3.   Place the trout onto a baking sheet and season with salt. Brush on some egg white before sprinkling the nut mixture all over the egg whites and pressing down.

4. Drizzle with some oil and bake the trout for 20 minutes to cook through before serving.

Ginger Tenderloin

Ingredients:

Pepper
Olive oil (1 ½ tsp.)
Sliced garlic cloves (1)
Pork loin (1 ½ lbs.)
Salt
ginger (1 tsp.)
sour cream (1 Tbsp.)
thyme
Dijon mustard (1 ½ Tbsp.)

Directions:

1.   Start this recipe by turning on the oven to 450 degrees. While that heats up, bring out a bowl and stir the salt, thyme, ginger, sour cream, and mustard together.
2.   Make small slits in the pork loin and then slip the garlic into the slits. Brush with the oil and add some pepper and salt.
3.   Heat up a skillet on the stove. Add the pork loin and let it brown on all of the sides.
4.   Now add on the mustard mixture and then move the pan you are working with over to your oven. Leave it inside the oven for a bit so the pork can cook through.

5.   Give this some time to cool after done with the oven and slice the pork a bit before serving.

Shepherd's Pie

Ingredients:

Pepper
Worcestershire sauce (2 tsp.)
Beef broth (1/2 c.)
Shelled edamame (2 c.)
Beef (1 lb.)
Minced garlic cloves (2)
Chopped onion (1)
Olive oil (1 Tbsp.)
Cauliflower florets (1 pkg.)
Salt
Cheddar cheese (1/2 c.)
Egg yolk (1)
Sour cream (2 Tbsp.)

Directions:

1.   Heat up the oven to 350 degrees. Fill up you're pot with a bit of water. Throw in the cauliflower and allow it to boil for a bit to become soft. Drain out.
2.   In a skillet, heat up some oil before cooking the garlic and onion inside for 5 minutes. Take the beef and

add it to a big skillet. Allow it to cook until the lumps are gone and the beef is brown.

3.   Take the edamame and throw in with the beef to cook. Stir the broth, pepper, salt, and Worcestershire sauce in as well. Move this over to the baking dish.

4.   Use an electric mixer and whip the cauliflower with the salt, egg yolk, and sour cream. Spoon this on top of the meat and then top with some cheese.

5.   Bake for 25 minutes and then serve warm.

Veggie Chili

Ingredients:

Pinto beans (2 cans)
Salt
Cumin (1 tsp.)
Oregano (1 Tbsp.)
Chili powder (1 Tbsp.)
Minced garlic cloves
Chopped celery stalks (2)
Chopped onion (1)
Chopped mushrooms (1 ½ c.)
Bell peppers (2)
Olive oil (1 Tbsp.)
Diced tomatoes (1 can)

Directions:

1.   Bring out a pan and heat some oil on high. Add the garlic, celery, pepper, onion, and mushrooms
2.   Cook these together to help the vegetables to soften. Then add in the salt, cumin, oregano, and chili powder.
3.   Allow these to cook for another 5 minutes. Add in the tomatoes and the beans and bring all of this to a simmer.
4.   Allow the chili to cook for another 30 minutes before serving.

Potato Salad

Ingredients:

Pepper
Chives (2 Tbsp.)
Hearts of palm (2 cans)
Olive oil (1 Tbsp.)
Minced garlic clove (1)
Dijon mustard (1 tsp.)
Lemon juice (2 tsp.)

Directions:

1.   Bring out a big bowl and whisk together the lemon juice, garlic, and mustard. While whisking, add in the oil a bit at a time.
2.   Then add in the chives and the hearts of palm. Toss it all around to combine.
3.   Season with a bit of pepper before serving.

Red Bean Mash

Ingredients:

Pepper
Cilantro (3 Tbsp.)
Salt (1/4 tsp.)
Vegetable broth (1/2 c.)
Red kidney beans (1 can)
Minced garlic cloves (3)
Chopped onion (1)
Olive oil (1 Tbsp.)

Directions:

1.   Bring out a pan and heat some oil. Add in the garlic and onion and let these cook until they are soft which takes 7 minutes.
2.   Add in the salt, broth, and beans and then bring to a simmer. Cook for another 5 minutes.
3.   Take the pan off the heat and stir in the cilantro. Use a potato masher to mash this into a puree.
4.   Add some pepper and then serve warm.

Baked Ricotta Custard

Ingredients:

Cinnamon
Vanilla (1/4 tsp.)
Half and half (1/4 c.)
Egg white (1)
Egg (1)
Sugar substitute (1/4 c.)
Cream cheese (4 oz.)
Ricotta cheese (3/4 c.)

Directions:

1.   Take out a bowl and use your electric mixer to beat the cream cheese and ricotta until creamy. Add in the sugar and beat until combine.
2.   At this time, add in the egg, vanilla, egg white, and half and half to mix until well blended.
3.   Move this mixture over to 4 prepared ramekins and then place these into a baking dish.
4.   Add some hot water into the baking dish to about an inch and then place into the oven.
5.   Turn the oven on to 350 degrees and let the custard cook for 45 minutes. Take out of the water bath and cool down before serving with some cinnamon.

Chapter 5: Recipes for Phase 2 of the South Beach Diet

Egg Frijoles

Ingredients:

Salsa (1 c.)
Beaten eggs (4)
Tortillas (4)
Cayenne (1/8 tsp.)
Pinto beans (2 cans)
Dried oregano (1 Tbsp.)
Minced garlic cloves (3)
Chopped onion (1)
Olive oil (1 Tbsp. and 1 ½ tsp.)

Directions:

1.	Bring out a skillet and heat up some oil on it. Add on the oregano, garlic, and onion, stirring a few times to make the onion soft.
2.	Add the cayenne and beans and then simmer, stirring a few times to make the beans warm and flavorful, which takes around 10 minutes. Cover and keep warm.
3.	While these are cooking, warm up the tortillas. When there is a bit of time left with the beans, take out

another skillet and heat up the rest of the oil. Add the eggs and scramble them for 5 minutes.

4. Divide the beans between the tortillas and top with salsa and eggs. Roll up and enjoy.

Oat Muffins

Ingredients:

Chopped walnuts (2/3 c.)
Salt (1/4 tsp.)
Cinnamon (1/4 tsp.)
Baking soda (1/2 tsp.)
Baking powder (1 ½ tsp.)
Pastry flour (1 ¼ c.)
Rolled oats (3/4 c. 2 Tbsp.)
Buttermilk (1 c.)
Vanilla (1 tsp.)
Beaten egg (1)
Canola oil (1/3 c.)
Brown sugar substitute (1/3 c.)

Directions:

1.   Turn on the oven and let it heat up to 425 degrees. Prepare a few muffin pans.
2.   In a bowl, combine ¾ cup of oats with the buttermilk and let it soak for at least 30 minutes.
3.   In another bowl and add in the flour, baking soda, salt, baking powder, and cinnamon. Slowly add in the walnuts.
4.   In another bowl, stir in the vanilla, egg, oil, and brown sugar. Slowly add in the oat mixture and then the flour mixture until they just start to combine.

5.	Divide this between the muffin cups and then sprinkle the rest of the oats over the muffins.
6.	Bake for 15 minutes and allow some time to cool before serving.

Eggsadilla

Ingredients:

Pepper Jack cheese (2 oz.)
Tortilla (1)
Pepper
Salt
Beaten egg (3)
Olive oil (1 tsp.)

Directions:

1.   Bring out a skillet and heat up the oil. Add the eggs and then reduce to medium.
2.   Scramble the eggs until they are cooked, which will take 2 minutes. Move to a plate and season a bit.
3.   Wipe out the pan and add in the tortilla, cooking on each side for just a few seconds to warm through.
4.   Top half the tortilla with cheese and then with eggs. Fold the other half over and cook for another minute before serving.

Thai Shrimp Soup

Ingredients:

Asian fish sauce (2 tsp.)
Chili garlic sauce (2 tsp.)
Tomatoes (2)
Shrimp (1 lb.)
Coconut milk (1 can)
Jalapeno pepper (1)
Sliced ginger (1)
Sliced scallions (2)
Lemon juice (4 Tbsp.)
Chicken broth (4 c.)

Directions:

1.   Bring out a pan and combine the pepper, ginger, scallion whites, lemon juice, broth. Take this up to boiling. Then turn down the heat and simmer.
2.   Stir in the coconut milk, fish sauce, garlic sauce, tomatoes, and shrimp. Return this to a simmer and cook for another 3 minutes.
3.   Remove the pan off the heat and divide this between 4 bowls. Sprinkle on some scallion greens and serve.

Roasted Tomato Soup

Ingredients:

Vegetable broth (1 c.)
Olive oil (1 Tbsp.)
Pepper
Salt (1/4 tsp.)
Oregano (1 tsp.)
Basil (1 Tbsp.)
Peeled garlic cloves (4)
Diced onion (1)
Tomatoes (2 ½ lbs.)

Directions:

1.   Turn on the oven and let it heat up to 425 degrees. Place some parchment paper on a baking pan. Arrange the tomatoes onto the pan and then scatter some garlic and onion on it.
2.   Sprinkle on some pepper, salt, oregano, basil, and garlic. Drizzle a bit of oil on top.
3.   Bake these inside the oven until the dish is done, or around 40 minutes. After this time, take the mixture out of the oven and move to a blender. Add in ½ cup of broth.
4.   Puree this until it is smooth. Move this over to a pan and then stir in the rest of the broth. Bring to a simmer and let it heat up before serving.

Turkey Sausage Soup

Ingredients:

Chicken broth (3 ¼ c.)
Escarole (1 head)
Minced garlic clove (1)
Salt
Rosemary (1/2 tsp.)
Chopped onion (1)
Olive oil (1 Tbsp.)
Turkey sausage (8 oz.)

Directions:

1.   Coat a saucepan with some cooking spray and then add the sausages. Reduce the heat a bit and then brown on all sides for 10 minutes. Move to a cutting board.
2.   Add some oil to the pan and heat it up. Add the salt, rosemary, and onion and allow it to go six minutes.
3.   Throw minutes. Cut the sausages in half going lengthwise and then into pieces.
4.   Add the escarole to the pan, going in batches, and then stir to make it wilted. Add broth and sausage and bring to a simmer. Cook another two minutes and serve.

Florentine Soup

Ingredients:

Chicken broth (3 c.)
Cubed cream cheese (2 oz.)
Spinach (1 pkg.)
Chicken breasts (2)
Pepper
Salt
Sliced garlic cloves (2)
Chopped onion (1)
Olive oil (1 Tbsp.)

Directions:

1.   Bring out a pan and heat the oil. Add in the pepper, salt, onion, and garlic. Allow this to cook together for seven minutes.
2.   Throw the spinach and chicken and stir for a minute before adding in the cream cheese. Stir this until it is melted.
3.   Now add in the broth and bring it to a simmer. Keep cooking until the chicken can cook through before serving.

Stuffed Chicken Breast

Ingredients:

Salt
Chicken breast (4)
Pepper
Basil (1/2 tsp.)
Minced garlic clove (1)
Chopped sun dried tomatoes (2)
Feta cheese (1/3 c.)
Olive oil (2 tsp.)

Directions:

1.   Preheat the oven to 425 degrees. Bring out a bowl and combine the basil, garlic, tomatoes, and cheese. Season with some pepper and then mash it together with the fork.
2.   Butterfly the chicken and then open up each breast and spread with some of the feta mixture.
3.   Close the breast with the filling and press the edges together to seal it up. Season with some pepper and salt.
4.   Bring out a skillet and heat some oil on the stove. Add in the chicken and cook to brown on both sides, about 2 minutes each.
5.   Move the skillet and place inside of the oven and then just let it cook to finish up the chicken.

Chicken and Soba Noodles

Ingredients:

Vegetable oil (1 tsp.)
Sesame oil (2 tsp.)
Soy sauce (1 Tbsp.)
Salt
Red pepper flakes (1/2 tsp.)
Ginger (1 tsp.)
Sliced garlic cloves (3)
Scallions (4)
Chicken breasts (1 ½ lbs.)
Soba noodles (4 oz.)
Lemon juice (2 tsp.)
Water (2 Tbsp.)
Button mushrooms (6 oz.)
Sliced Napa cabbage (1 head)

Directions:

1.   Bring out a pan and bring water to boil. Cook the noodles until the are done.
2.   While this is cooking, bring out a bowl and combine together the salt, pepper flakes, ginger, garlic, scallion whites, and chicken.
3.   Drain out the noodles and move over to a bowl. Add in the sesame oil, soy sauce, and scallion greens.
4.   In a skillet, heat the vegetable oil. Cook the chicken for about 5 minutes and then move to a plate.

5. Now add the water, mushrooms, and cabbage. Cook until the vegetables wilt. Add the chicken back in and cook for another minute.

6. Toss with some lemon juice and serve.

Herbed Turkey

Ingredients:

Chopped parsley (4 Tbsp.)
Italian bread crumbs (1 c.)
Milk (2 Tbsp.)
Beaten egg (1)
Pepper
Salt
Minced garlic clove (3)
Turkey cutlets (1 ½ lbs.)
Button mushrooms (1 lb.)
Olive oil (1 Tbsp.)

Directions:

1.   Coat the turkey with some of the garlic and salt and pepper. Bring out a small bowl and whisk the milk and egg. Spread out the bread crumbs on a big plate.
2.   Dredge the turkey into the egg mixture and then through the bread crumbs on both sides.
3.   Use some cooking spray to cover a skillet and cook the turkey in batches until crisp. Sprinkle with some parsley and then cover with foil to keep it warm.
4.   Add the oil as well as the remainder of the garlic and parsley along with the mushrooms into your skillet. Cook for 5 minutes.
5.   Move the turkey to the plates and then top with some mushrooms before serving.

Halibut and Vegetable Ragout

Ingredients:

Chopped tomatoes (2)
Pepper
Basil
Salt
Crushed garlic cloves (2)
Chopped onion (1)
Olive oil (2 tsp.)
Halibut fillet (4 pieces)
Butter beans (1 can)
Peas (1 c.)

Directions:

1.   To begin this recipe, bring out a pan and heat up some oil. Add the pepper, basil, salt, garlic, and onion.
2.   Reduce the heat and let it cook for 4 minutes. Stir your peas inside of this along with the tomatoes and allow it to warm up.
3.   Now add in the beans and cook for another 2 minutes. Take the pan off the heat.
4.   Place the halibut into a broiler pan and brush with some oil. Broil until it is opaque, which would take about 8 minutes.

5.   Divide this among four plates and serve the fish and the ragout together.

Shrimp and Scallop Bake

Ingredients:

Chopped parsley (1 Tbsp.)
Lemon zest (2 tsp.)
Lemon juice (2 tsp)
Olive oil (1 Tbsp.)
Pepper
Salt
Minced garlic cloves (3)
Shrimp (3/4)
Sea scallops (3/4 lb.)

Directions:

1.   To start this recipe, bring out a bowl and combine the garlic, shrimp, scallops and season with pepper. Toss this around until the seafood is coated through.
2.   Bring out a skillet and heat up the oil. Add your premade seafood mixture and cook it for about 4 minutes.
3.   Move over to a serving bowl and add lemon zest and juice. Sprinkle a bit of parsley and serve this warm.

Stir-fry with Beef

Ingredients:

Water (2 Tbsp.)
Snow peas (6 oz.)
Minced garlic clove (1)
Sliced onion (1)
Sliced green bell pepper (1)
Olive oil (1 tsp.)
Pepper
Round steak (1 ½ lbs.)
Soy sauce (1 Tbsp.)

Directions:

1.   Take the steak with some pepper and salt. Bring out a skillet and coat with some cooking spray.
2.   Add the steak inside and cook for about 4 minutes and then move off the heat. Move the steak to a board and give it 5 minutes to cool before you slice it.
3.   Inside this pan, allow the oil to get warm before throwing in the pepper, garlic, and onion, cooking these for 5 minutes.
4.   Add in the water and peas and cook until the vegetables are soft and let it cook for 5 minutes.
5.   Uncover the pot and add in the soy sauce. Cook this for another 30 seconds. Add the sliced steak and toss it around a bit. Serve it warm.

Lamb Stew

Ingredients:

Rosemary (2 tsp.)
Peeled and smashed garlic cloves (4)
Chopped onion (1)
Celeriac (1 diced)
Diced carrots (2)
Pepper
Salt
Lamb (1 ½ lbs.)
Olive oil (3 tsp.)
Peeled tomatoes (1 can)
Dry red wine (1/3 c.)
Tomato paste (1 Tbsp.)

Directions:

1.   In a pan, heat up some oil and add in the lamb. Cook for about 6 minutes so that the lamb is browned on the outside. Move this over to a plate.
2.   Add in the rest of the oil to the same pan and add in the rosemary, garlic, onion, celeriac, and carrots.
3.   Cook, stirring until the vegetables will start to brown. Add the tomato paste and cook another minute before adding the wine and cooking some more.
4.   Add in the tomatoes and their juice before bringing this to a simmer. Allow this to be a bit cooler and cook for a bit to let everything get nice and warm.

5.   Return the lamb and cook to heat it through before serving.

Barley Risotto

Ingredients:

Pepper
Salt
Parmesan cheese (1/4 c.)
Pearled barley (1/2 c.)
Sliced onion (1)
Olive oil (2 tsp.)
Chicken broth (3 c.)

Directions:

1.   Bring out a pan and bring the broth to a simmer. When it warms up, take it off the heat.
2.   Meanwhile, bring out a big pan and let the oil get warm inside the pot. Throw the onion and barley inside as well and stir it to combine.
3.   Turn the heat down and then stir so the onion turns softer and the barley is toasted for five minutes.
4.   Add a third of the broth and bring this to a simmer and cook for another 12 minutes until it is absorbed.
5.   Repeat with some more broth, slowly adding in the rest of the broth. Your cooking time will be about 50 minutes total.
6.   Take the pan off the hit and stir in the pepper, salt, and Parmesan. Serve this warm.

Sweet Potato Chips

Ingredients:

Pepper
Salt
Italian seasoning (1 Tbsp.)
Olive oil (2 tsp.)
Sweet potatoes, sliced (2 lbs.)

Directions:

1.   Bring out a big bowl and toss the potatoes together with the pepper, salt, Italian seasoning, and oil.
2.   Spread out a bit of this onto a baking sheet and turn the oven on to 400 degrees.
3.   Bake the chips for 10 minutes and then use a spatula to turn them over and cooking another 7 minutes. Serve these warm.

Chapter 6: Recipes for Phase 3 of the South Beach Diet

Classic Burger

Ingredients:

Sliced red onion (1/2)
Sliced tomatoes (1/2)
Lettuce (4 leaves)
Dijon mustard (2 tsp.)
Swiss cheese (2 slices)
Pepper (1/4 tsp.)
Salt
Ground beef (3/4 lbs.)

Directions:

1.   Heat up a grill and let it be warm. Bring out a container and allow the beef to mix together with some pepper and salt and then mold into patties.
2.   Grill the patties until they are done as much as you would like. Layer on the cheese slices and cook for another minute to allow the cheese to melt.
3.   Take two leaves of lettuce and layer on different plates and then the patties. Spread the mustard on top and before topping with the onions, tomatoes, and lettuce before serving.

Steak Wraps

Ingredients:

Whole wheat wraps (4)
Salt (1/4 tsp.)
Lime juice (2 tsp.)
Sour cream (1 Tbsp.)
Chopped tomatoes (2)
Romaine lettuce leaves (2)
Flank steak (1 ¼ lb.)
Peppers (1 Tbsp.)

Directions:

1.	Take the peppers and rub them all over the steak. Place this into a bag and let it marinate for about an hour.
2.	Turn on the broiler and then place the steak inside to cook for 5 minutes on both sides. Take the steak out and let it cool on a cutting board for 5 minutes. Cut into slices.
3.	Take out a bowl and combine the salt, lime juice, sour cream, tomatoes, and lettuce.
4.	Warm up the wraps in the microwave for 30 seconds and then lay them out. Add the steak and the rest of the ingredients and then roll up tight to finish.

Conclusion

The next step is to get started on this diet plan. We spent some time talking about the different phases that are involved in this diet plan (remember that there are three to help you learn how to lose weight and keep it off) and you will be able to get started with the first one as soon as you are ready to get started. Then you can move through the rest of the phases at your own rate, depending on how much weight you have to lose and how quickly it comes off.

The ideas behind the South Beach Diet are simple and they are there to help you to lose weight efficiently, but you still have to put in some of the work. This is not a quick plan that will be easy and you can lose weight in your sleep, but if you follow the advice that is in this guidebook and use some of these recipes to help you out, you will find that losing weight can be easier than ever before. When you are ready to finally lose that weight that has been sticking around for years, make sure to pick up this guidebook and learn about the South Beach Diet.